When We Kneel, We Learn

When We Kneel, We Learn

A Look at Caregiving Through the Lens of Faith

by

Kayla Morgan Dudley

RESOURCE *Publications* • Eugene, Oregon

WHEN WE KNEEL WE LEARN
A Look at Caregiving Through the Lens of Faith

Resource Publications
An Imprint of Wipf and Stock Publishers
199 W. 8th Ave., Suite 3
Eugene, OR 97401

www.wipfandstock.com

PAPERBACK ISBN: 978-1-6667-0721-2
HARDCOVER ISBN: 978-1-6667-0722-9
EBOOK ISBN: 978-1-6667-0723-6

DEDICATION

To my parents and grandparents, who have always provided for me. To my sweet friends, who have loved me just the way I am. To my mentors, who both shape and reassure me when I am confronted with the questions of life. To Laura Ellis-Lai, who advised me with such gentleness and who gave me confidence in my work. She would always remind me that I am the author of this book, and she respected my beliefs even when they differed from her own. To Elisabeth Olszewski, who encouraged me to write this book. Elisabeth not only freely offered to read and edit this piece before publication, but she freely offers in many areas of her life that others will never see but I will appreciate for eternity. To Adam Castillo, who joined me in seeing work as something we "get" to do rather than something we "have" to do. To my precious residents, who have changed my life for the better. To the Lord, who is my foundation, and from whom I pray all things flow.

Table of Contents

TABLE OF CONTENTS

Caregiver Terminology

Transfer: The act of lifting a resident in order to move them from one position to another, usually accomplished as a one-person task but may require two people or a gait-belt for assistance.

Brief: A padded undergarment that is worn by residents that are incontinent to prevent messing.

Memory Care Unit: Another term for the Alzheimer's and dementia unit; a locked unit that houses residents living with memory loss.

Med-Passer: Staff member that administers medication to the residents, usually working alongside a caregiver.

Pager: Button that each resident has in order to call for help/assistance from staff.

When We Kneel, We Learn: how kneeling is an act of humility in the face of understanding, forgiveness, building relationships, and loving the elderly: A book for those who want to provide better care for the elderly; A book for those who yearn to know more about such a beautiful generation; A book for those who long to see that empathy is reaped where understanding is sowed; A book for those who desire to know how love reaches its full potential through experience; A book for all.

Tender Touches

The little girl touches the
Grandmother's arm
"You don't know how long I've waited to be known,"
The Grandmother smiles
Eyes weary from wonder
Why do her children
Never visit
"They think they want you around,
And then they realize they made a
Mistake,"
She tells the young girl
"Shh," bow-in-her-hair girl responds
Wishing she could give
More than just a
Tender touch
Of empathy
Sometimes words are insufficient to heal
What someone feels
Within
The girl does her best to . . .
Reassure that . . . That is *not* the case
But is it?
As indicated by how infrequently
Younger people
Visit the *nursing homes*
Elderly
Put away
Forgotten

Their own brains deceiving them
The cruel hand of dementia
Grandma and Grandpa
Work all their lives
And then expected to be idle
In a home
Foreign to what they've known
The last seventy years
What an individualistic society
We live in
Where the elderly
Are *forgotten*
Tender touches
Tender words
There is such a want for these things
The job opportunities
Are great
To love
Grandmothers and Grandfathers
Not our own blood
But of our own soul
Grandmothers and Grandfathers
Longing to be known,
Go.

Introduction

IN THIS PIECE OF creative nonfiction, I have put together an autobiographical work about my experience in a caregiving facility over the expanse of two years. I touch on numerous topics, such as finding avenues to include the past hobbies of the elderly into their current reality as well as particular approaches to take when working with those living with Alzheimer's and dementia. The richness of what this work gave me while pursuing my degree was so profound that I knew I had to be a voice for my elders. Being an English major, I have always said that I want my words to speak life and to speak it abundantly, and writing a book is the best way that I knew how to do that for the geriatric population. This memoir is aimed directly at those interested in caring for the elderly, with quotes, stories, and insights gained from my personal experience and, most importantly, through the lens of my Christian faith. Whether you are a college student volunteering at the local nursing home, you plan to make a living out of this work, or you anticipate having a beloved relative in a care facility, this book is for you. In fact, if you are a human and interested in deeper relationships, this book is for you. The time will come in life for most of us to have our turn at caregiving. Maybe one day you will be staring into the eyes of a mother or father who once held you, and it will be your turn to hold them. I hope that this book is a blessing.

The bonds that I have created with this generation have contributed to an awe and appreciation for my elders, an insight into their wisdom, a perspective on life that is familiar to my old soul, and a spirit that resonates with my own. Because of them, I now have a lesson on loving, living, and servanthood. I have cared for former artists, nurses, park rangers, supervisors, and missionaries. The cycle of life comes around full circle: people care for others, and then they eventually need to be cared for. My job is to make sure that by the time the people that took care of *me* and my generation reach the age when they need to be cared for, they are getting the same love that they gave in return . . . *And then some.* As my executive director once told me, the best generation is dying. When I expressed to him how that was a sad statement, he told me: "We shouldn't be sad. We are the ones that are taking care of them. We should be happy." What I have gained from the elderly will be with me for the rest of my life. In this way, the generation will live on. Stories keep memories alive and shape the way one views the world. **I hope my story will tell theirs.**

About the Author

It is in the sufferings of this present life that my soul has beckoned me to draw nearer to the Lord. My faith is a lens through which I see the world, and the Bible keeps me accountable on those days where loving people just doesn't seem like it's something that I *want* to do. If there were to be any inspiration in connection with this memoir, my Heavenly Father is the building block on which it stands. If it wasn't for Him, I would not have the integrity it takes to keep striving toward a heart more like His. I would not consider a cheerful countenance and a kneeling servant's heart to be such high callings on my life. I would not have had the supernatural energy on my six a.m. shifts to be a light for my residents. I would have permitted a complaining, dispassionate attitude toward my job and those within my care. God is the one who gives me the motivation to be truthful; the one who convicts me to be genuine. God is my reason for kneeling before those in need, as He kneeled down to wash His disciples' feet … and as He kneeled under the weight of the cross for me. One night, I had the thought that the Lord said to me, "Take care of my flock," and I said, "Show me how, Lord. Please help me."

There is nothing that I have found to be more fulfilling than loving God and loving others. My hope is that people will always feel like they have a soft place to land with me and a seat at my table. Therefore, I leave you with this, my precious readers: please take a seat at my table and be fed. I pray that these words show you the heart of the Father, as well as the heart of His elderly children, of whom He says: "Even to your old age and gray hairs, I am he, I am he who will sustain you. I have made you and I will carry you; I will sustain you and I will rescue you" (Isaiah 46:4, NIV).

Chapter One:

Empathy

Dear Reader,

My hope for this chapter is that it encourages love before bitterness and understanding before judgement, particularly when it comes to those elders that are more difficult to care for. I pray that amidst the grind of this work, caregivers do not become individuals who are on autopilot, monotonously attending to their tasks. This chapter is intended to shed light on how crucial it is to stop for conscious contemplation within this job and to sacrifice your time to truly get to know the individuals within your care. Most importantly, I hope that you will put yourself in their shoes . . . and in the shoes of all those who you meet and are called to love. We would want others to show the same mercy toward us.

(Scribble 1) Empathy for Audra

The first time I stepped foot into Miss Audra's room, I knew that she was very ill. A head bald with affliction, a pale shadow cast across her skin, an oxygen mask dangling from her face. The sight of sickness can often be a scary one. However, if everyone's sickness was as physically obvious as Audra's, perhaps we'd have more compassion for one another. It didn't take long after meeting Audra to realize that she was a woman who was prone to lashing out, getting easily frustrated, and executing sarcastic comments on a regular basis. One day in particular, I was confronted with a situation in which Audra was treating me unkindly and began to raise her voice while I was trying to help her. Although I became frustrated and felt like crying, I was able to utilize the message of empathy and put it to practice. I reminded myself of how she must have felt: a three-time cancer survivor and hardly able to do anything for herself after being such an independent person throughout her life. No wonder she was irritated! Wouldn't most of us be? From this perspective, I could show Jesus' example. It was my job to uphold His kingdom testimony, so I had to continually nudge pride out of the way and let love cover all sins. It was so releasing to walk away from the situation, come back with a clear mind, and have a normal conversation with her once again. As scripture says, "A gentle answer turns away wrath" (Proverbs 15:1, NIV). I don't think Audra ever realized that she had hurt me by her actions. However, showing her love in return was so much more rewarding than letting her hurts and humanness get in the way of the compassion that I had the opportunity to demonstrate to her. This perspective was a much lighter burden to bear, both for me and my residents. This mindset allowed me to feel sympathy and sorrow for the person that was hurting me, knowing that they, too, were affected by the brokenness of the world. I knew that if I allowed bitterness to be planted, it would grow and do more harm than good. I knew that what started out as an irritation would fester and germinate into hatred in the long term if I allowed it to. I learned that relationships are like a mirror which allows us to be confronted with our true intentions, sinful tendencies, and the potential to work on those faults with humility rather than pride. I was to have empathy for my residents as I sought to understand them, all the while knowing that I had never been in their shoes or walked their path. I would never truly know the extent of what they went through in their childhood or the trials that they faced when others weren't watching. My job was not to know, because that was God's job; my duty was to seek to understand in the midst of uncertainty, to refrain from judgement, and to fight against my own sin. I would want others to show the same mercy toward me.

Jesus Himself demonstrated the ultimate example of mercy when He died for those who crushed Him with the weight of their sins.

On another occasion, Audra audibly made a sarcastic comment pertaining to no one caring about her well-being. It was later on in the afternoon that I was able to help her into bed for a much-needed nap. She asked me if I could wake her up in about an hour so that she wouldn't miss an event that the other residents at the facility were participating in. Almost an hour went by, and I returned to her room and reminded her of why I was waking her up. It was then that she got the biggest smile on her face, leaving me pleasantly startled, and reached out to take my hand in her own. I was instantly reminded of her comment that no one cared and awakened to the realization that she just wanted someone to think of her. She wanted to not be forgotten about amidst her sickness; to not be confused or left out of the loop; to not feel lonely. She wanted to be normal and included. The root cause of her complaint was that she felt excluded, and that came out of her mouth in sarcasm because she was hurt. I learned that when I seek to understand the roots of an issue, I can then work toward being more empathetic for why people act the way they do.

You see, resident Audra helped me to see the raw consequences of doing the right thing in the midst of the pressure to do the wrong one. The wonderful thing about this is that I found myself in awe at what was happening within me as a result of putting this to practice. Humans are so encouraged when they see the result of their kindness in their own experience. It's just a matter of displaying that kindness in times when it is most difficult to do so in order to discover the benefits that it reaps in the latter end. Empathy is seeing the best in another individual amidst their *worst* moments and then being in awe when that person later demonstrates the *best* side of themselves.

When I sat down with Audra to converse, to ask for advice, and to look at her as an elder rather than someone who needed to be cared for, I saw a woman that radiated confidence, was riddled with wisdom, and was sure of her knowledge. I learned of a woman that was a nurse and a teacher. I was met with messages that I needed to hear from someone as blunt as she. I was looking at a mentor. You see, when we kneel, we learn. When I took the time to give her my attention, sitting in a chair eye-level with her wheelchair, I was a student in her classroom. At a time when my career choices were on the line, she looked me dead in the face and said matter-of-factly, "Life is not made of absolutes. What you choose to do with your career is not something you have to do for the rest of your life. If you don't like it, you can change it later. It's not the end of the world."

Talking with Audra, I was met with a woman of faith. A woman that told me that growing old is inevitable. God gave us a certain number of years to figure out how to live and whose lives we are going to touch. Growing up is a choice; we can choose to be young at heart or we can choose, in her words, to be "smudgy" and "mugged." Sometimes God uses the people you would least expect to give you the message that you need the most, and somehow that makes the very message all the more valid. Audra told me that the only way she could have gone through what she did was with God; it wasn't something she could have handled on her own.

Audra was, by far, one of my most difficult residents. Simultaneously, she was also one of the ones that encouraged the most character growth within me. It's quite funny how that works: the most difficult trials are the ones that grow us the most if we have a heart that's open to growing. The relationships that cause the most tension can also cause the most spiritual development. The Audra that almost made me cry, was the same one that I found myself hugging. The hardest resident was also one of my biggest lessons.

I found that if I ever want to learn anything from others, I surely need to understand the art of forgiveness. In the face of people failing me, I cannot close off my heart to the value that they can still contribute to my life and the world around them. I humbled myself to understand that people hurt me because they are hurt, and I am called to forgive them because we are all sinners and misunderstood. People have a tendency to disregard others when they mess up, but Jesus calls me to release both myself and those around me through the art of forgiveness, compassion, and mercy.

Audra taught me that I never know who will need that forgiveness seven times a thousand, and I can be their cushion of grace. I can be the one who sees that they have a lot more to offer the world than most people realize.

(Scribble 2) Shoes of Another

It was not long before I picked up on the annoyance Harold brought out of my coworkers and the other residents. Whether it be his long, drawn-out conversations, his inability to hear very well, or his complaints about not having gravy on his rice or cranberry sauce with his turkey. The truth is though, I always had a soft spot for Mr. Harold. I adored the man with the high-waisted pants and a belt over his big, round belly. The man that was unsteady on his feet and nearly fell backwards when I tried to give him a high-five one day. The man who had this huge, teethy, quirky smile, and who loved to tell stories. I would see him at the dinner table talking away to his table mate, who would be sitting beside him, turned away with his eyes closed. One day, I witnessed him with a group of residents who were all playing a trivia game and getting increasingly annoyed each time they had to repeat what they said to him. Yet, *there he was*. Harold was *himself*, seemingly un-phased by others' opinions.

If there was anything that Harold taught me in the time that I was blessed to spend with him, it was what it means to be misunderstood. As a Presbyterian Minister, he was used to having a whole pulpit to talk on. He had engaged in the art of storytelling as his career, with a crowd of listening ears awaiting his teachings. He was considered outspoken at the assisted living center, but only because it was his job to be outspoken throughout his life. He was used to having the stage, and now he was encouraged to be silent. I learned that it was important for me to push myself to imagine how oppressing that must have been for him. To imagine engaging in a conversation, having a thought bubble up that begs to be expressed, and having to push that thought back down the throat and swallow it whole. Harold was taught to speak his whole life, and by the time he was over ninety years old, he was encouraged to cease speaking. Such is the case for many of our elderly today.

Harold expressed to me more than once that he was lonely after having spent years of his life falling asleep beside his wife. He was used to having someone to express his ideas to, someone to give him personal companionship, and someone to supply him with the beneficial human luxury of physical touch.

By disciplining myself to become knowledgeable about my residents' pasts, I could better understand how to comfort them in the present. Once I sought to understand him, Harold was no longer merely Harold: he was Minister Harold, husband Harold, and father Harold. He was so much more than just his name; he had a history that had consequently affected and shaped the rest of his life. Because of this, I could position myself to listen when he had something to say, with the vast amounts of knowledge that he had acquired over the course of his lifetime. I could challenge my-self to give him a hug in order to help soothe the ache of his wife's absence. I learned that intimacy in the form of communication, touch, and proximity is so significant in the lives of the elderly, especially when considering the significant losses that they have endured throughout their experiences. However, this presents it-self as a challenge amidst the hustle and bustle of being a caregiver. To *make* the *time* to truly have empathy for another is a virtue in and of itself, chiefly when there is a ticking clock, a list of duties to accomplish, and residents paging for help in-between. The longer that I worked in the field, the more pressing the temptation became to offer a simple, "I'm sorry," and to carry on with the day's tasks. There is this dangerous desensitization that comes with familiar-ity in the workforce as well as in other areas of life. There were numerous times when I could have easily slipped into the mindset of there being nothing else that I could do for a particular resident. This would have been a cop-out in the midst of preoccupation and selfishness. It was in those moments where I worried that I would not get off on time if I spent the extra ten minutes with a resident, or those moments when I was thinking about what I wanted to do after work. The less I lived in the present with the beautiful individual in front of me, the more likely that the quality of care they were receiving was going to be negatively impacted.

There were daily tests of character in the position of a caregiver. Oftentimes, the challenges were tensions within myself. No one else would have known about them, but I would have to live with myself at the end of the day. For example, one time I was getting a resident changed for bed. I had just put a brief on her and was transporting her to bed when she pooped in the *new* brief during the transfer. Already having spent an excessive amount of time with that resident, I had a mental conflict in my head about whether to change her again or to leave the responsibility to the next shift. Being convicted, I decided to change her again in bed and – believe it or not – one of the brief straps TORE this time. Yes, sometimes in life everything goes wrong. I learned that all I can do is my best, and then it's my turn to give myself grace. Rather than changing the resident again, I just taped the side of the brief that was torn and called it a day. I try to go the extra mile, but I am not faultless. That very fact gives my perfectionistic self a much-needed reality check. My deficiencies have allowed me to acknowledge that I have to rely on the Lord and His Word day after day. I can be a great caregiver and servant, but only the Lord can be a *perfect* one.

I had to sacrifice my time to *get to know* Harold and my other residents before I could attempt to understand them. I learned that there is a fine line between the word sympathy and the true act of sympathizing with another human being. You see, people love the *thought* of compassion. However, compassion is such a necessary characteristic to have in this cruel world that individuals become indifferent to it. The news is constantly airing bad reports, whether it's pertaining to an active shooter in a school or a child that has been diagnosed with terminal cancer. By the time a person has an individual placed in their life that needs empathy, they can naturally be apathetic to their pain; sorry for their trial, but altogether un-feeling. It is only when I die to myself and my wants that I can rejoice with those who rejoice and weep with those who weep (Romans 12:15, ESV). It is only when I learn people's stories and take the time to ask myself how it must feel to be in their place that I can be moved by the art of compassion. It requires the act of ceasing activity and engaging in contemplation. In such a busy society that prompts me to work and live on auto-pilot, I have learned that I must go against the grain and be a conscious, thinking being. Starting with people who are misunderstood, such as Minister Harold. Oftentimes, the things that annoy me in other individuals are areas of their life that I fail to understand. I must be careful not to disregard the roots of people's issues, and therefore discard their whole being. Instead, I can seek to comprehend their story and be enlightened in discovering why it is that they do the things they do.

(Scribble 3) Revelations From Lilith

The most truthful statement I could ever make about being in a caregiving facility is that I do not know how it feels to be the recipient of such care. Not yet; not in this young body. I do not know what it feels like to be separated from family, to be in a foreign environment, to have a life that is now merged with the lives of numerous other individuals my age. I can try to empathize; attempt to relate based off of similar life scenarios such as my college experience, but I am not eighty years old and having to start anew. Ninety years old and being prompted to form new habits in a fresh environment. One-hundred years old, bed-ridden, with a family that can only visit occasionally. Frequently, *at best*. Aging brings with it limitations, and those limitations are unique from my own experience.

Lilith was a resident full of revelations; a beacon of insight into the minds of my elders. She was a ninety year-old German woman with eyes that could hardly see and a racing mind that continuously prompted her to walk around the facility. Back and forth. Back and forth. Into other residents' rooms and even out of the facility altogether before she was caught by one of her peers. One day, I had the honor of speaking to Lilith's son, who informed me that she had survived World War ll and lived off of molasses and potatoes for nearly a year. If that wasn't already telling of the fact, he said that Lilith had a hard youth.

I was able to sit down and talk with Mrs. Lilith one day when she first arrived at the facility. She was an intelligent soul with lots of self-awareness mixed in with her confusion. She told me that she was someone that "tells it like it is," and that her children sometimes didn't like that. However, she insisted that she had been behaving lately. Lilith really did think that her time at the facility was a vacation. In fact, she was very concerned about her fifteen year-old cat, "Sandy," that *just happened* to jump in the car with her on the way over. I explained to Lilith that her apartment was where she would be living from now on. She responded, "Here? It's ugly!" in her crackly, feminine accent.

Lilith was honest about many things, but perhaps one of the most heart-wrenching aspects of her honesty were her unfiltered expressions about the isolation and loneliness she was feeling within. Referring to her children, she told me: "You get old, and then you're always in their way. They think they want you, and then they realize they made a mistake."

As a caregiver at an assisted living center, I found that there was one thing that I would always lack: the ability to devote an abundance of time to each resident. When pagers and to-do lists beckoned me, Lilith stated, "Don't leave me, I just need some empathy-like." Sometimes, I had to leave. Never was it fun.

Even whilst enduring the effects of dementia, Lilith was still able to communicate how discombobulated she felt within. At one point, she vocalized, "I don't like this place." When I asked her why, she responded with, "It's tricky." Such a simple, straight-forward statement that would represent her state of mind during the months that followed. Lilith went on a journey of exhaustion. She would walk and walk, wearing herself out daily and not getting adequate rest. Eventually, Lilith was moved to the memory care unit of the facility and would often display how restless she felt. She would make comments such as, "I'm so nervous." She would ask, "How do we get out of here?!" One time, she even had to sit on her hands to alleviate her anxiety. Movement was her way of coping, and her and I would go on walks outside to unleash some of the energy that was built-up in her body.

Sometimes, it doesn't matter how nice a caregiving facility is. A foreign place is a foreign place. Separation from family is still separation from family, and quality cannot heal that wound like relationship can. Soul connection will always be more important than material resources, and that is why a caregiver's job is so essential at its core.

In which you can ask yourself:

1. What would it feel like to pursue a life-long career in a culture of hustle and then be expected to remain idle in your last years?

2. What would it feel like to be taken out of a place you called home and be put into a nursing facility at the age of eighty+?

3. How can caregivers use the sacrifice of their time and empathy to attempt to understand the depths of uncertainty that the elderly around the world feel on a daily basis?

Chapter Two:

Love And Learning
from Those We Care For

Dear Reader,

My hope for this chapter is that the giving hearts of these residents will inspire a tenderness in yourself. May you be humbled – as I am – to know that we can learn from the very ones that we are called to serve. May you see that the endurances that these individuals have survived through produced great faith and compassion within them. Here, I emphasize the forms of intimacy that deepen the quality of care that the elderly receive by their caregiver(s). I hope to demonstrate that there is a caregiver/client relationship that surpasses job descriptions and enters into the depth of loving and being loved.

(Scribble 1) I Love You is a Common Phrase: Dahlia and Edith

> *"Religion that is pure and undefiled before God the Father is this: to visit orphans and widows in their affliction, and to keep oneself unstained from the world" (James 1:27, ESV)*

Some may say that hatred is the opposite of love, but I would argue that isolation and loneliness are equally as opposed. From their place in their reclining chairs, where they lived and where they slept, I heard the phrase echo from both Dahlia and Edith's lips: "Please don't leave me." Unfortunately, I eventually *would* have to leave them and tend to the next resident, not knowing if they would get the proper care until I saw them again.

As the Lord calls me to visit the widows in their affliction, I must at least attempt to understand the *depth* of that affliction and what that visit means for those heavy hearts. At twenty, I did not want to forget what it felt like to be sixteen. At twenty, I also wanted to acknowledge that I did not yet know what it feels like to be eighty. In order to carry others' burdens, it is helpful to realize what those burdens *are*. I was to put myself in the shoes of the elderly in the nursing facilities. I was to ask myself what kind of care my aging mother and father would deserve, and proceed to treat the elderly with that same type of care. When I saw my residents, I was to see children of God with immeasurable worth if I truly wanted to love them to the best of my ability. This meant that no matter what they did or said, it couldn't be taken to heart and therefore affect the quality of care that they were receiving. I met residents who were former nurses, teachers, missionaries, artists, volunteers, and veterans. People who once freely gave of themselves for others and deserved the same treatment in return. The elderly can often be looked at as helpless, but I have grown to understand that they are individuals who were once independent now stripped of their freedom. Women who used to cook for their families who now need to be cooked for. Men who worked with their hands whose hands are now crippled from a stroke, arthritis, or are shaky from Parkinson's. People who contributed greatly to the world around them but can no longer put together coherent sentences as a result of age wearing down their minds. Some individuals who used to see their family frequently and now are lucky if they even get a visit. Isolation and loneliness deprive humans of feeling love; we are beings that were made for companionship. As one of my residents, Thomas, once told me, "I'm afraid to go anywhere, cause memory is merely a word in the dictionary nowadays, seems like . . . I used to have a house and a car, and now I have none of it."

Dahlia was undoubtedly one of my favorite residents that I ever had. With her colored sunglasses to match every outfit, her long gowns, and her scarves, she was a character, to say the least. She was my buddy. I would often creep into her room right before I started work, kneel, and give her a hug in her recliner, where the biggest and sweetest smile would burst out across her cute face. I did this because I loved her, and I actively loved her because I made it a point to form a bond with her that stimulated that very love. We can always say we love someone, but it is the *effort* that is put into loving that allows it to reach its fullest potential. Love is an action and a choice. Feelings are like undulating waves that come and go.

One day, Dahlia had a peculiar look on her face, to which I asked her, "What's wrong, are you okay?" She merely shook her head, so I asked again: "What's wrong?" She replied, "I'm just so happy you're here." Sometimes, just being *there* for another individual makes all the difference in the world. With the open invitations to her fridge, her genuine smiles, her talks of George Bush (who, come to find out, she knew personally in her younger years), the sweetest voice you've ever heard, and her friendship, Dahlia was someone who will live on in my heart for the rest of my life. She was more than a resident: she was the giver and recipient of love. Before I would leave her room, I would often tell Dahlia, "Don't let the bed bugs bite," and she would respond with, "I'll bite em' back." I used that line with my other residents long after she passed, and I could see that something so simple made them *happy*.

Dear Edith was another one of my favorite residents, who I would often find slumped over asleep in her recliner. She had puffy white hair, a tender and sweet North Carolina accent, and a precious smile that was an outward portrayal of her loving soul. To care for her was to be welcomed into her room as if I was a part of her family. The only time she would come out of her room was when her relatives would visit her or when she was taken to the dining hall to eat. When I would draw near to Edith, she would reach for my hand and bring it up to her cheek to rub it against the skin. I would crouch down and hug her, to which she would respond, "I love you, darling." She would rub my arms as if I was her child. Edith taught me the importance of physical touch for the elderly who are often deprived of such skin-to-skin contact. This is something that one will come to realize is on a person-to-person basis. One individual's comfort level will not be someone else's. Therefore, it is necessary to first form friendships, bonds, and intimacy in order to evaluate what each person needs in order to feel loved, as well as the boundaries that it would be disrespectful to cross.

One thing is for sure: Dahlia and Edith taught me that "I love you" is a common phrase for those who have hearts that are open to giving and receiving such love.

(Scribble 2) Kitty and Clara

Working with the elderly has taught me about the delicate nature of a giver's heart. In the face of a generation that has seen and endured much, I witnessed the results of such endurance in the form of faith and compassion. I have seen residents take the time to push their wheelchair-bound friends from the dining hall back to their rooms nearly every single day. I have seen them take interest in each others' lives, spend time together, and keep each other company as if they were a family. They would ask questions of concern when one of their peers was missing or in the hospital. They recognized the absence of others and therefore understood the value that *every* person's presence adds to a community. The elderly are not perfect; they are human and flawed like the rest of us, but being around them has made me a better human.

My resident, Greta, would demonstrate Christ-like love by handing out little peppermints to each person she passed by. She would make sure to stop with her little walker and put out her hand containing the red and white treat. She brightened days through her tiny acts of service. After she passed away, Greta's daughter donated a tub of those peppermint candies in her honor. We never know how much the smallest deeds can lift up a weary spirit. It is not as much about the candy as it is about the heart that went into it. When Greta served, her actions told others: "I care about you."

Audra once told me about the beautiful soul of her mother. She said that she would go hungry sometimes to ensure that Audra and her father had food. It was in stories like these that I uncovered the sacrifices that had to be made by a generation that lived out the years of The Great Depression. I began to understand why it was essential to form compassion amidst such hardship. I learned how these struggles shaped my residents' character. Throughout my life, I have heard that if we want to gain wisdom, we should spend time with our elders, and I have seen that come to life through my work. Just by opening my mouth to ask life-questions, I could receive profound advice from those who had already experienced it for themselves. With multiplied years, the elderly have faced the ups and downs of life and learned to embrace both joy and suffering. How did they live through it? Just ask them.

When I think of Kitty, I think of tenderness. I think of a gentle voice, like that of a counselor, accompanied by a warm smile. I think of someone who would look me directly in the eyes when talking with those beautiful blue gems of hers, without haste or intimidation. I think of someone who was soft and kind. When I would take care of Kitty, I would often be met with a woman who would reach down, pick up her bucket of chocolates, and tell me to help myself. "Take more," she would say, as I always felt guilty for taking more than one sweet. One time she would offer cake, another time she would make me try her buttermilk . . . other times it would be the ice cream bars in the fridge.

Noticing Kitty's giving heart, one day I confronted her about it. The statement she said that her daughter told her is imprinted on my heart to this day: "Momma, no one could ever accuse you of being selfish." What an accurate depiction of Kitty.

I like to think of Mrs. Clara and I's relationship as a god-wink in each others' lives. Although our time together was brief, that's all it took. The first time I met her, she and I successfully flooded the bathroom as I gave her a shower, she apologized profusely as I mopped it up with about 6 different towels, and we later proceeded to joke about it. It was quite the scene. That night, Clara told me how shy she was to go to the dining hall with everyone else because of her shaking disease. This petite, adorable little old lady, as sweet as she could be, ashamed of something she couldn't control. Afraid of people's judgement. Yet, when I looked at her, I couldn't imagine someone not liking her. I tried to encourage her not to worry about something she couldn't help, and that it's about the heart (something us humans know, but so often forget). It wasn't but days later that she adamantly insisted that I split her salad with her, asked me to take yogurt or pudding from her fridge, and told me where the grocery bags were in her room! She basically wanted me to go shopping! Talk about a giver. It was no time before we were sharing I love you's. I've come to realize that, oftentimes, the elderly may see their children, their grandchildren, and their loved ones in the form of their caregivers. In the absence of blood relatives, caregivers become their comfort and company amidst the loneliness that they experience, and that is a beautiful thing. Little did my residents know, they were often my comfort as well. Sometimes, we think we are a blessing, when we really are the ones being blessed in this life.

In which you can ask yourself:

1. What are the implications of our elders seeing us as their family? What kind of weight does that carry for the integrity you should uphold as a caregiver?

2. What does it mean to have a respectful intimacy with the elder within one's care? What does it look like for that elder's individual personality, background, preferences, and boundaries?

3. What kind of heart does it produce in us when we realize we are being blessed by the very ones we think *we* are serving?

Chapter Three:

The Sacrifice of Our Time
and Investing in Others

Dear Reader,

My hope for this chapter is that it will shed light on *why* we care for others and the suggestion that the word *care* in *caregiver* conveys. I hope it demonstrates that time is a sacrifice, and there is not a greater sacrifice than investing that very time in the Lord and His creations. I hope that these stories encourage you to look at those within your care as individuals that you can include in your daily life.

(Scribble 1) More Than a Warm Body

My resident, Ollie, was a quirky fellow, with collared shirts tucked into his business pants and toes busting through the holes at the tips of his old shoes. His crooked-tooth smile could light up a room, and he derived much joy from those who truly cared for and loved him. He was a character with a timid countenance and a heart for justice. One day, when I walked into his room, he made me giggle at the sight of a chunk of his hair, normally plastered neatly against his scalp, sticking straight up in the air. When I told him about it, he sweetly said, "I'd a fixed my hair if I knew you were coming."

Something will always stick with me that Ollie vocalized one day: "They treat me like a warm body." Time and time again, he would express to me how caregivers would walk into his room with a straight face, wouldn't dare crack a smile, would do their job and then leave. It impacted his life, but it wasn't the kind of impact that left a positive mark. I could only imagine how vital day-to-day interactions would be if I spent 90 percent of my life in a two-bedroom apartment. Such was the life of Ollie, as well as many other elderly today.

Now, as someone who lived out how unrelenting the job can be, I dearly sympathize with caregivers. I endured days where pager after pager went off, the demands were high, the gratitude from those being cared for was low, and the staff were few. It was moments like these when caregiver burnout could occur, and it was in these times that I *had to* take a step back, take a break, and ask myself *why* I cared for others. It was these moments that were a true test of character. The mind was confronted with two options: caving under the pressure of the responsibilities or truly putting my residents' needs first. The answer demonstrated whether I did my job to be recognized and thanked by residents and staff or to make a difference. Whether I did it for people to see or for God to see. Whether I did it just to get the job done or to self-sacrifice and willingly lay down my life for those around me. My calling was (and continues to be) putting aside my pride, my selfishness, my reputation and my "need" for recognition. Galatians 6:10 reminds me: "So then, as we have opportunity, let us do good to everyone, and especially to those who are of the household of faith" (ESV). Matthew 6:3 reminds me: "But when you do a charitable deed, do not let your left hand know what your right hand is doing" (NKJV).

A home-health nurse at our facility once said something that I found to be very insightful: "In order to prevent caregiver burn-out, do not take your job with you. Do what you can at work and know that you did all you could do, but don't take it home. You can help them (the residents) to the best of your ability, but you can't hurt for them or stay up all night worrying about them because you will get burned out. You can only do what you can when you are there."

I got to thinking: How could I be a source of strength for someone if I crippled myself with their pain? Perhaps carrying someone's burdens looks a lot like putting myself in their shoes for a moment but *not dwelling there*. Maybe it looks like empathizing with one's weaknesses and drawing from my strengths to lift them up. Maybe it is about putting others before myself even in the midst of my own fleeting sufferings. If I stay up all night worrying about the ones I love, I will not have the energy to help them when it is needed. I learned that this idea applies to any realm of work: if people take their cares home with them, they will consequently be unfair and neglectful to the rest of the individuals in their lives. It took me a long time to discover that I cannot save people. I can do what is in my human ability and then proceed to leave the rest in the Father's hands. Anything less is hindering my own ability to serve from a full well.

From my time as a caregiver, I learned that people don't just want to be waited on, they want to be *invested* in. They want someone to show them that they are more than just a warm body or a number. This requires immense selflessness – especially in the midst of pressure. I learned that it would do me well to continuously realize that time is a sacrifice. I learned that I make time for the things that I *want* to make time for in this life. I intentionally choose how I spend my moments as well as the quality that those moments will be. As a caregiver, I sometimes had to choose between giving a resident optimal care and therefore sacrificing the demands of the job, versus giving a resident average care and caving under the pressure of the job's other responsibilities. As sad as it is, such is life, isn't it? Sometimes, I had to be willing to selflessly risk getting in trouble for the sake of doing what was right. I could take the weight of my burdens out on those around me, or I could smile amidst the strain. I could choose to merely do what was in my job description or to go the extra mile. I could choose to just give my residents their daily showers, or I could take the time afterwards to give them a foot massage. I could just deliver room service, or I could take the time to ask someone how their day had been or if there was anything else I could get for them. Looking at Jesus, He didn't just eat with the disciples; He washed their feet. He even did this for Judas who would soon betray Him. Jesus *invested time* in those He cared for. He was intimately acquainted with the likes, dislikes, hobbies, joys, and hurts of those He loved.

From *investing in* Ollie, I came to know that he was from Germany and could speak the language, almost got married to a German girl before his brother called him back to the states, never had any children, loved avocados, tomatoes, and fish, was in the military, had been living with heart disease for years, had much insight to share about history, and loved giving the longest hugs. These things may seem like random discoveries, but I learned that it is a gift that we can give to another when we allow them to share with us the joys, burdens, and life experiences contained within their heart. We may or may not gain something from listening . . . but they gain much from feeling *heard*.

One time, I had a resident named Ada who was in assisted living for a very short time while her family was on vacation. I had a simple job with her. She stayed in her room, and I merely needed to deliver and pick up her room service. That would have been easy. After all, humans tend to be enticed by the easy. However, I asked her how she was adjusting to the facility and let her know that I hoped she felt welcome. This allowed for a certain amount of vulnerability to be unlocked, and Ada proceeded to tell me that she was lonely and nervous. Over the course of the next few days, I asked her if she had adjusted yet, to which she replied, "That's so sweet of you to ask." Her comment baffled me because it reminded me of how easy it is *not* to ask, yet how essential it is to *do so*. Before our time together ended, Ada told me: "You've taken such good care of me." Yet, all I had done was go a little bit past the easy. Ultimately, I found that the best way to love my residents was to make sure that they knew I truly cared for them *as an individual*, rather than just the duty that I was accomplishing in "caring" for them.

(Scribble 2) Not Just a Resident, a Friend

There is a hidden chest of delicate and tender treasures to be found when a caregiver ventures in and opens the vulnerable box of friendship between them and their residents. There is something sweeter than honey to be tasted when the avenue is opened to a greater reality beyond the basics of care. There was something deeper and longer-lasting that I found when I allowed myself to love well enough to *know* the residents that I was loving, meanwhile allowing them to know *me* all the same. There was something life-changing about such a surrender to relationships. It was no longer just a client-caregiver dynamic. It was so much more beautiful than that. There was something about the way that I could go home and write the precious words of my residents in my journal to remember for years to come. Something in the way that they felt comfortable enough to share parts of themselves beyond what I deserved to hear as their employee. Almost magically, there was no longer a separation between being a caregiver and a confidante. The vulnerability of love merged the two together in harmony. It was no longer a: "Hi" when I walked into a resident's room. It was a: "Hi, Kayla!" It was no longer a: "Hello, I'm here to get your trash." It was a: "Hi, Ollie. How are you?!"

A friend is a storyteller. One day, my one-hundred year-old resident named Isaac told me about the leaky spigot at his old home that contributed to the growth of tall daisies. He told me that his wife's favorite flower was the African violet, and that she had one in every window. In that moment of sharing, his tender heart was my own. The depth of preciousness that the memory held in his soul was one that made my own soul more precious by hearing about it. The delicate simplicities of life.

A friend is a caregiver. One day, Mrs. Kitty told me, "Come here," from her place in her recliner. Holding my hand, she said, "Your hands are dry, you need lotion," and proceeded to make sure that I used some of hers.

A friend is a life-sharer. When I got my wisdom teeth out, my residents knew about it. They wanted pictures when I moved into a new apartment. They knew about my life, and I knew about theirs.

A friend is a chosen family. It was Charlotte calling me her adopted daughter. It was Emily telling me that I had to take care of myself when I was working after getting my wisdom teeth removed. It was 102 year-old, sweet and brutally honest Lucinda telling me that I was trying to do too much. In a way, my residents were my grandparents. It was important for me to allow myself to have the mindset that *they just care* rather than feeling as if they were trying to tell me what to do. These ladies were speaking to me as a grandmother would. Indeed, one of my dear elderly friends requested that I call her *grandma,* expressing that I was closer to her than her own grandkids. She told me of how she and her husband used to have a grandson but that he never connected with her anymore. She seemed to be so hurt about it and reminded me to never forget about my own family.

In which you can ask yourself:

1. We all understand that people are more valuable than objects. Therefore, why is it so easy to put the object of job responsibilities over the bonds created with those within one's care?

2. What would it be like to feel as if you were one amongst the masses in a nursing facility and that the caregivers always had something or someone else on their mind?

3. How can a caregiver ensure that each resident is seen and feels uniquely valued?

Chapter Four:

Finding Familiarity

Dear Reader,

My goal in this chapter is to encourage your mind to think about the passions that are familiar to those within your care and incorporate those very practices into their day-to-day life. If the passion cannot be completely restored due to the restrictions of aging, I encourage you to think about simplified versions that can be utilized to brighten the lives of your elders. Idle time truly can be the devil's playground, and leaving the elderly alone to their thoughts can foster a variety of mental disturbances in the form of anxiety and depression. I hope that through this chapter, you learn the significance of productivity in human beings who were created to *create*. Most importantly, I hope that you are moved to awe that you are able to give back to the very ones who served others throughout their lives.

(Scribble 1) Finding Familiarity

One day, resident Edith was continuously looking out the window and had mentioned going for a walk. Considering that I had the extra time, I was able to meet her need and take her for a stroll a few times outside. It was beautiful to see how the small things were so significant to her: the bird feeders and the flowers on display. Come to find out, Edith used to garden. When the elderly find aspects of life that resonate with them, it brings them back to their personal interests and provides a sort of familiarity to their day. It comes down to caregivers making time to understand their elder's past hobbies and incorporating aspects of those interests into their daily agenda.

Similarly, I was in awe when I witnessed music therapy at work in individuals' lives, specifically those living with Alzheimer's and dementia. As the elderly gathered around to listen to songs from their youth, their mouths instinctively began singing the lyrics. It was a beautiful display to see amidst the loneliness, uncertainty, and confusion that can come with aging, disease, and being in an environment where people must rely on others for care. I witnessed my memory care residents perk up and sing along as they sat in a circle around the activity coordinator who played guitar and sang to them. I listened to the types of songs that were selected; ones that resonated with the elderly and allowed for them to reminisce on their younger years: Amazing Grace and tunes by Elvis Presley. In fact, one of my residents would randomly belt out "God Bless America" on a frequent basis. One day, he even got all of the other residents to sing along. Boy, was it a sight to see. It is moments like these that are precious to me and will continue to be treasures to look back on. It is often a difficult task to get those in the advanced stages of memory loss to say much at all, but music was the gem that awakened my residents' minds and hearts. Somewhere deep within, these songs were imprinted on their souls, and they preserved an aspect of their lives amidst the many other aspects that were fading away.

I have seen the mastery of finding familiarity and how it was used in the lives of former artists through simple art classes. These individuals were no longer able to exercise their raw talent, but they could engage in a hobby that comforted them through the utilization of their natural passions. These activities were merely presented to them in a simpler format. My resident, Maggie, was given coloring books due to her love of the past-time. Similarly, some residents were encouraged to help fold laundry in the memory care unit or bake yummy desserts to spur them to embrace their inner homemaker, caregiver, and nurturer. It was women like Georgia and Penelope that these tasks resonated with. Georgia was a stay-at-home momma in her youth that absolutely adored her children. She would sometimes talk of taking her little ones to the pool when they were younger with a picnic of tuna fish sandwiches. It was evidently a fond memory for her nurturing soul. Penelope, on the other hand, was one of the hardest working residents that I ever had, all the while living with a very advanced stage of dementia. She could be found doing chores, such as rinsing dishes in the sink or pulling chairs out from under the dining room tables so that she could sweep. It was duties like this that she took upon herself and were evidently so good for her to engage in, as they corresponded with the kind of personality and lifestyle she was used to. Sometimes, finding familiarity is merely allowing the elderly to be who they are and watching them embrace their natural inclinations.

I learned that I could incorporate various activities into the lives of the elderly and those around me when I took the time to learn and understand where their loves lied. I discovered that life is about challenging myself to fall in love with the hobbies of another and joining them in the participation of such hobbies *for their sake*.

(Scribble 2) The Remedy to Idleness

A wandering mind can quickly become a house for depression, anxiety, and immense loneliness in the lives of the elderly. One of the greatest disservices the younger generations can do is to constantly leave elders alone to their thoughts. Human beings are made for companionship, no matter the age.

It was not a rare occurrence for me to hear my elders speak out about their boredom. One resident of mine, Thomas, that suffered from chronic memory loss, frequently made the statement, "Slow day at black rock, huh?" Another woman named Nora talked about how she was bored to death, and Charlotte and Moses regularly wanted to be "put to work." While these were the few that had the voice to express themselves, there are many elderly that are not so fortunate. Whether it be because they are living in smaller facilities with less funding for activities or because they do not have the capacity to coherently speak, their needs are muted. Even whilst working at a facility that was large enough to be able to give residents many choices for engaging events, it was still difficult to always meet the wants and needs of everyone within our care. Therefore, it is essential to change the activities so that they grow with and cater to the community at the time. As my executive director, Wallace Reynolds, said, "You change activities to meet the residents' needs. You don't just say that 'this is the way it's always been.'" In other words, the environment must adapt to the community it contains. Furthermore, it is in the heart of service that one goes the extra mile and confronts the individual interests of the residents. People should not merely be seen as a collective mass, but rather, as individuals *within* a community.

One day, as I was working the front desk during the COVID-19 pandemic, one of my residents with the onset of dementia, Moses, approached the counter in front of me. His old body was ready for the manual labor that only his younger body was qualified to perform. He stated the following: "This is a request, can you do that? There's a huge field out there in the back (of the facility) that my wife and I look at when we eat. I would love to get out there and plow that and plant all kinds of fruits and vegetables. So tell someone there's a nut in here that wants to work." This is the kind of boredom that may arise among individuals that are not ready to settle into a life of solitude. In society, specifically in western culture, someone is expected to work their life away in a haste and then retire into stillness. Sometimes, the brain does not catch up to this sudden jolt of change in activity, even at the age of ninety! It just doesn't seem fair for a head full of anxious ambition to be turned away. Moses wanted to move his body like he used to, and no one should turn that down if he is still able. The problem that presented itself during the pandemic was that it was prohibited for the residents to go off of the facility grounds. This rule was put in place in order to prevent the spread of the virus. However, the quarantine regulations were not only foreign, but forgotten, in the minds of those living with moderate memory loss. Moses and Thomas asked multiple times if they could leave the facility, to which I would reply that they could only go for walks around the building and sit on the porch. In situations like these, words are meaningless if there is not a beneficial alternative in place. If there are no ways to supplement for the unmet needs of a resident, they will *find* ways to attempt to satisfy themselves. This could potentially cause harm to their own bodies or to the bodies of those around them. Despite the conversations that I had with Thomas and Moses, both of them decided to walk by themselves to Walgreens, where they were found by one of our staff on duty. Additionally, Moses took another trip across the highway and ended up being picked up by a kind stranger who graciously drove him back to the facility.

There is a very human and natural independence that makes its appearance in the elderly when they have to take matters into their own hands. While this is not a negative thing in and of itself for those who still have their memory, it can be detrimental for those who are beginning to struggle with memory loss. If boredom does not create problems, it can cause self-isolation, depression, or a loss of purpose in the elderly population. It was my job as a caregiver to find creative ways to listen to the residents' needs and meet those needs to the best of my ability. One day, one of my residents was visiting the memory care unit and was eager to leave. To keep her hands and mind busy, I rolled her up to the dining table and told her that I really needed her help folding clothes. She executed the task with precision and was much better at folding than I was. Of course this was the case; she had been a wife and a mother!

One of the sweetest people that I have ever had the pleasure of meeting was my resident, Charlotte. To know her was to love her. To pour her a cup of coffee was to be met with a kiss on the hand. She could normally be found in the facility's community room with an outfit that matched from her head to her feet. If your eyes met her face, a wink or a warm smile would be sent your way. If you asked her how her day had been, she would often reply, "Honey, every day is a good day that you can get up and move around." Charlotte's personality was benevolent, and her perspective was one of great gratitude for life. She was the kind of woman who would not hesitate to lift a finger if she saw a need; even within her ninety year-old body, she did not doubt her ability to help another. In fact, one day I spotted Charlotte pushing wheelchair-bound Grace into the community restroom. Already en route with another resident, I made a mental note to come back downstairs to check on Mrs. Grace. When I did so, I was met with the most startling, funny, and sweet sight! Opening the bathroom door, I came upon Charlotte helping Grace pull her pants down on the toilet. After smiles, a laugh, and a hug given to Charlotte because of how cute and sweet she was to play caregiver, I took over the job. Before walking out of the bathroom, she made sure to tell Grace that if she ever needed anything, to let her know . . . and proceeded to blow her a kiss.

One day, I was taking mail to be distributed to the residents' rooms. Charlotte had this very concerned look on her face and said, "Honey, you can't get all that by yourself." I got a cart to put all of the mail in, but she persisted in asking if I needed help. She expressed to me that she was *very bored*. This was the perfect opportunity to utilize idleness in a productive way for both the residents and the staff. It probably appeared very strange to my coworkers to see little Charlotte tagging along with me to hand out mail. However, most efforts of servitude have to be embraced with the willingness to go outside of the box. One thing I've learned is that if I feel awkward about something potentially wonderful, I should embrace it. Within facilities, when time is short and staff are few, it is essential to formulate creative, innovative ways to cater to the whole community. Sweet Charlotte travelled both floors with me and delivered mail under residents' doors. At one point, I told her, "This is kind of fun, isn't it?" to which she replied, "Oh yes, honey. Very." She was such a good little helper and so quick on her feet. As a school teacher for thirty years, she told me that her students used to tell her that she was walking too fast for them at recess. In fact, Charlotte and I would sometimes go for walks together after work. I began to refer to us as the "bullet ladies." This would make her break into laughter. She would often tell me, "You little rascal," with a chuckle.

Charlotte would always speak fondly of her teaching days, never uttering a bad word about her students. When I would ask her what grade level was her favorite, she would tell me, "Honey, all of them." During my quiet times at work, Charlotte and I would work on a puzzle together. This not only provided joy by mere engagement in the activity but the fact that we could sit side by side in one another's company. I am a firm believer in the idea that *presence is a form of servitude.*

I think there is this idea that society imposes on people that acts of grace toward our fellow human beings must be extravagant. However, service should be a mode of life in all of its forms. Charity is not something to make a show of, nor is it something to be done infrequently. It is to be the method that I live by, in its subtlety and gentleness. Love does not beg to be noticed, because it realizes that helping others is its expected calling. It is the act of staying after work because one truly cares about how the residents are doing behind their closed apartment doors. It is learning which genre of books a resident likes, how they met their spouse, and what their favorite hobbies are. It is about bringing devotionals and encouraging books to someone who just moved in and is having a hard time adjusting. Charity is subtle; it is the soft hum beneath the noise of the world. It is what one does when those around them are busy with daily tasks.

Charity is my coworker and dear friend, Elisabeth. She is simple and yet full of more love than the most complex showcases. Her heart asks not to be seen, yet it is more obvious in its simplicity and humility than it ever would be in its boasting. Elisabeth asked me to join her off the clock to spend time with sweet Charlotte one evening. My friend brought in one of her necklaces that had broken to show Charlotte how to restring it. This may seem like a mundane chore, but it was not so for an elderly woman who would always ask for something to keep her hands busy. As Elisabeth and I sat in Charlotte's room and worked on our own projects, the tender soul repeatedly told us, "I am just so thrilled you girls would come and spend time with me." She allowed me to sit on the floor of her quaint, tidy apartment and flip through the photo album full of retirement notes from those she worked alongside. They were awe-inspiring to read; they moved me to feel honored that I had the privilege to get to know and care for someone who was highly esteemed by so many. My role was to give back to her what Charlotte had given to others. Each paragraph below presents a note from someone who knew Charlotte. The following offers a snippet of what it was like to walk alongside her in her younger years, which beautifully explains how she habitually blossomed into the person she was in her old age.

> *Throughout our marvelous, wonderful years together, you have inspired me to write many delightful thoughts in my journal. These thoughts have always been a great blessing in my life, for God has blessed my years with our friendship.*
>
> *How long has it been? It's been just another day, another day for you to touch the hearts and lives of an uncountable number of students, faculty, friends, family, husband, two sons, two daughters-in-law and four grand-children. Your 'just another day' has been a lifetime for us. We've all experienced a lifetime of your love and giving, giving of yourself. Your giving has been and continues to be an example for all of us.*
>
> *From one perspective, twenty-nine years is a long time. From another, it is all too brief. Today is on the side of brevity. It is hard to know how profoundly you impacted the students at the academy as well as others in the academy family. It is safe to say that people all over the world are better because you were their teacher. We are grateful for what you are and the work you have done.*
>
> *You are an aberration in a self-serving world! I have tried to imitate you, and therein lies my genuine reason to miss you. My mentor is now gone; your protege is on his own. So, I hope that I have a portion of your grace and style to perpetuate. I will miss your physical presence, but your emotional and spiritual presence will be with me forever. THANK YOU MORE THAN YOU WILL EVER KNOW!*

Lastly, *Thank you . . . for being you, a miracle of grace in my life.*

In which you can ask yourself:

1. What hobbies bring joy to your life? How would it feel if you could no longer participate in them?

2. What are the past-times of those within your care? If you do not know, what are some creative ways to ask? How can you incorporate versions of those hobbies into their present reality?

3. Can you imagine what your elders were like in their younger years and how they contributed to the world you now live in? How can you give back and honor their servitude?

Chapter Five:

Relationships and Companionships

Dear Reader,

My hope for this chapter is that the elderly demonstrate a mature and realistic display of love, relationship, and companionship; one that endures through conflict and is rooted in commitment and covenant. A love that places more value on choice over feelings, and shows that our views on love do not have to constantly change with the times. It is beautiful and healthy to learn from the generations before us.

(Scribble 1) Charlie and Beatrice

Love is often emphasized in the Bible: "Love your neighbor as yourself," "For God so loved the world," "Love covers over a multitude of sins," "Love is patient, love is kind" (Mark 12:31; John 3:16; 1 Peter 4:8, 1 Cor. 13:4, NIV). Yet, perhaps love cannot be felt to its utter depths until it is experienced for what it is at its very core: unconditional. If God is love and God is perfect, He is the only one from whom we can receive that unconditional love that our hungry souls long for. However, as an individual that is made in His own image, I can yearn to love perfectly and strive to have that kind of care for another spirit as I follow after Christ's example. I can see God's love in the creations around me, see His work when I look in awe at nature, and *choose* to see the Creator when I look into the face of another human being. In spectacular moments throughout this life, I can even see hints of His unconditional nature echoed in the actions of those around me. These come as rare gems and remind me of how immensely my inner self desires for this kind of selfless, precious, and genuine care.

The first time I met Charlie and Beatrice, I met them as two separate bodies. The first time I met them *together*, I met them as a unit. Two united as one. A covenant relationship. Charlie's love said: for better or for worse, I will love her. This was the meeting I preferred, as it was more pure and magical than the best of love stories. They were better together.

It is firstly important to know Charlie and Beatrice's backstory. Beatrice was an incredible artist and dancer throughout her lifetime and was in the advanced stages of dementia when I had the chance to care for her. Charlie was living in the assisted living unit of the facility and would often come to see the woman in which he spent a life-time with. The woman in which he shared hundreds of memories with, raised children with. He saw her in her peaks, and now he would see her in her lowest of lows. Yet, he willingly did so. Oftentimes, Beatrice would resort to babbling, taking off her clothes in front of the other residents, and crying when we would wrap ourselves around her in a hug. Sometimes, the only way to get her dressed was to tell her, "Beatrice, let's put on your pretty clothes," because it would bring her back to her dancing days. In fact, her old costumes were splayed around her apartment in the memory care unit.

I was in awe when I first witnessed Charlie and Beatrice's connection. I remember that first day when he walked into the memory care unit, put his hands on either side of her face, and tenderly kissed her forehead. She would reach for him or say things that indicated the longing she had for his presence. Perhaps her heart remembered things that her mind could not, or maybe her brain allowed for faint traces of such an immense part of her life to be preserved. These things I do not know, but I do know the wonder that I felt when Charlie would sit beside her and hold her hand while they watched television or sat outside in the fresh air.

I think he knew that she couldn't understand what the screen was showing, nor could she embrace a nice day any longer. Perhaps he couldn't either, because when she passed away, Charlie said that he no longer had any reason to live. It was only months later that he followed her into heaven. I do believe that he died of a broken heart; one that no longer felt a reason to fight. Isn't that why we stay on this earth? We feel like we are needed, have a purpose to carry out, or see the necessity to stay strong for another? Charlie was staying strong for Beatrice. Eventually, his strength was no longer needed, so he released it and lost the fight.

I profoundly remember one day when I was sitting beside Charlie and Beatrice as they held hands, and he softly plucked off a leaf that had drifted onto her pants from a nearby tree. I began to ask him about her, and words of praise for his wife poured from his lips. Meditations that he had probably re-played in his mind naturally slipped out sweetly like honey. He began to cry as he explained how amazing she was, and yet she sat beside him completely unaware. That's something like unconditional love, isn't it? Love that is not able to be properly reciprocated; praising another without them knowing it; adoring someone so much that a negative word is dared not uttered; being so in love that it gnaws at the deepest recesses of your being? As Charlie left to go back to his own apartment later that day, I let him out of the locked doors. He couldn't help but slip in a few more words about his beloved wife as he teared up once more. He cared for her so deeply that he couldn't help but share her qualities with anyone who would listen.

If you ever walked into Charlie's apartment, you'd see Beatrice's beautiful paintings splayed around his room as vivid reminders of that peak at unconditional love.

(Scribble 2) Marriage

"I opened for my beloved, but my beloved had left; he was gone. My heart sank at his departure. I looked for him but did not find him. I called him but he did not answer" (Song of Solomon 5:6, NIV).

Before my pastor left this world at ninety years old, he told me to thank the Lord every day in my journal for my future husband. I stuck to that order almost religiously over the years. In my later teens into my twenties, I eagerly sought out insight about being the best wife I could be, preparing my heart for such a commitment in due season. I had had dreams of married life for the last few years. I often found myself watching sermons about relationships and Ted-Talks about love. Many times, I spent my nights watching soldiers coming home videos, pregnancy announcements, and long-distance couples meeting for the first time on YouTube. I would read books about what it meant to be a godly wife. I wanted to be the kind of spouse that could be utterly myself, and for that to be a blessing of joy to my husband. I wanted to keep singing and dancing around the kitchen and delighting in the Lord, and for that to be a light to the one with whom I chose to spend the rest of my life.

One delightful blessing of working with the elderly was the plethora of relationship advice that they had attained over the years and could therefore pass on to me. Talking of and witnessing the love between my residents gave me a realistic understanding about lifelong commitments rather than the false picture that movies and books had painted for me over the years. My residents gave me a tangible grasp of what *real* marriages look like. I learned that a purer form of love is the type that keeps pursuing even in the face of opposition, hurt, selfishness on the partner's end, and unfair responsibilities. Love will never be fair; it surely wasn't when Jesus sacrificed his life for us. I learned to *expect* a sacrifice rather than an easy match. I learned that everyone has their baggage, and that it's about choosing to love someone without measuring their amount of baggage against someone else's. Love in this life is going to continue being a struggle, and a 'perfect' partner won't be an exception to that. I now understand that a fairytale life isn't as conducive to character growth.

For my residents, real love bore underneath the oppression of life's many hurdles. It bore underneath illness, relocation, and even death. It continued on in the memory of its beloved for the sake of its own life still to be lived. Henry was one of these great bearers of such love. He was a resident in the memory care unit with a select number of stories to repeatedly tell. His stories were ones worth re-hearing simply because they made such an obvious impact on his life; they were glimpses of what he had left of himself to hold onto. Henry would often talk about his late wife with such passion, occasionally tearing up at the mention of her passing. He would say that "she loved her initials," and would spell them out for me: "B-A-D. Bad!" followed by a deep, throaty laugh. He sure did get a kick out of that. Henry was a jokester at heart, and anyone that was around him long enough could tell that he liked to maintain a lighthearted perspective on life. Often, when I would go into his room to pick up trash near the end of my shift, Henry would ask me in a gruff, humorous voice, "You gonna steal my trash?!" and then chuckle hysterically at my response. Henry was a sweet soul with a well of hurt deep in his heart. He missed his wife of forty + years. He missed their life together. He said that she was his dance partner, and that when she died, he stopped dancing. He said his family thought he was going to die, too.

The beauty of love is that it stretches beyond marital bonds and settles into something that can be referred to as companion-ship. Such was the case for Georgia and Henry. Georgia was the former stay-at-home mother in the memory care unit who often wore bright red lipstick, a wig, and a sweet heart on her sleeve. She made a wonderful companion for Henry, having lost her own husband to the cruelty of memory loss. Georgia and Henry would sit outside together under the balcony or sit inside holding hands. Sometimes, they would talk about life and death: both parts of the human experience. Other times, they would just sit there holding each other. Occasionally, humans just need the mere *presence* of one another. When Georgia took a nap, Henry took a nap. When he forgot that she was napping, he would look around the com-munity for her. Georgia wasn't Henry's wife and never would be, but they were a source of love and friendship for one another that was crucial for the quality of their remaining lives. They were each others' backbone and sounding board when no one else could be.

After Henry got sick and was sent out of the community for weeks to recover, he just wasn't the same upon his return. He began to sleep his days away, and his huge appetite reduced dramatically. Even in the midst of memory loss, Georgia didn't forget about her care and concern for Henry. One day after his return, he had been sleeping the evening away, and he finally came out to the dining table to eat. Georgia made sure to put on her wig and join him at the table, keeping him company and eating M&Ms and Reese's alongside him. When his energy was exhausted once again, she proceeded to walk him back to bed and tuck him in for the night. She would often give him a goodnight kiss.

Mr. Jack and Mrs. Hattie had a very similar bond to Henry and Georgia's. These two lived in the assisted living unit of the facility. With Hattie being someone affected by the onset of memory loss, Jack went from being a stranger to being a great source of support for her. Jack would guide her around the facility as she followed suit. They would watch movies together at night on her couch. He was her rock. When he left the facility, she would ask about "her husband," look for him, and was inevitably lost without his direction. It took a long time for Hattie to stop missing Jack. Sometimes, I would find her staring off into the distance with a sad look on her face. Unfortunately, his family was not open to them sharing even one last phone call in the wake of their separation and Jack's deteriorating health. It is stories like these that have taught me the significance of companionship in a marriage. There is something pure about being able to do life alongside another breathing soul.

If love were a mere feeling, it would surely perish under the weight of Alzheimer's disease. To see one's beloved endure such a drastic change in character guarantees that a spouse does not end up with the same person that they married. A disease such as memory loss does everything in its power to strip an individual of the very qualities that make them who they are. To watch that transformation from the eyes of a lifelong lover must feel something like betrayal. Irritability, confusion, loneliness, apathy, and sadness emerge in the wake of a tethered mind, which naturally affects the emotional health of one's spouse. Perhaps you cannot watch someone you love go through something so harsh and remain unchanged.

June was a woman in the Alzheimer's and dementia unit who was generally unresponsive. She could often be found with her eyes closed or rolling behind her head. A plump lady, her appearance consisted of short, baby soft hair and a tender face. The most activity June's day consisted of was being transferred from her bed to her recliner or wheelchair. Throughout COVID-19, her husband, Felix, was persistent about seeing the love of his life. If he couldn't see her in person, he was either FaceTiming her or holding her hand through the outside fence, with a chair pulled up next to her wheelchair. One time, he even came to see her through the window, and my coworker said that it looked like he had tears in his eyes. For their anniversary, my coworker and I set them up with a video-call. It was precious to see the way he interacted with his sweet June, especially in the midst of her not being able to reciprocate. On the occasions when she did open her eyes, he would make comments such as, "Look at your pretty blue eyes." After the call, we sent him a picture of his wife smiling, and he expressed how he loved us and conveyed his gratitude for us "taking such good care of her." Every little thing was special to him; every little thing that people so often pass up and take advantage of day to day was a blessing. As someone who has always cherished the minuscule details in life's corridor, this was a further indication of the significance in simplicity. It reminded me to be grateful when the time comes where I will wake up every morning next to someone who I *choose* to spend my life with. It reminded me that it is a *privilege* to love and give myself wholly, rather than a burden or an inconvenience. It reminded me to take note of the ways in which I want to cherish and bless my husband some day. To be grateful that he has eyes that still open, a mind that still works, hands that can still reach for my own, and arms that will hold me close. It reminded me to make his life easier whenever I can, even by things as arbitrary as putting toothpaste on his toothbrush in the morning before work or writing him a letter that he can read on the way out the door to lift his spirits. To let him know that I am proud of him . . . *just* as he is. There were so many privileges day to day that June's husband could no longer embrace, but his eyes for the little blessings gave him the strength to never give up on the pursuit of his wife.

One of the lessons that began to sink in during that summer of 2020, is that love is a constant test of an individual's character. I began to see love as an art to be continuously perfected within *myself*; a way to grow in acceptance of one's beloved; to allow them to be who they are and to love them for it. I began to see love as something liberating rather than restricting for the person within one's care.

In which you can ask yourself:

1. Are your thoughts, words, and actions building others up?

2. What does companionship mean for a human race that was not created to do life alone, and how can you grow to adore and respect those relationships among your elders?

3. What can you learn about love from those you care for, and in what ways has it departed from its intended nature throughout the years?

4. In what ways has love improved throughout the generations? What is love to you?

5. How must it feel for our elders to lose the very person that they did life alongside? How can you meet them in that hurt and serve in the broken places of their hearts?

Chapter Six:

Perspective/Supernatural Energy

Dear Reader,

My hope for this chapter is that it gives glory to God. I hope that it shows how my faith has shaped my perspective, especially when I didn't have the energy in and of myself to properly execute my tasks as a caregiver. Perseverance has enabled me to detach from myself and my wants in order to serve those that I am blessed enough to have in my path.

(Scribble 1) Supernatural Energy

There were those five-forty-five a.m. shifts where one of my residents would ask me how I had "that much energy" so early in the day. To this I would reply: "God gives me the strength." There were the days where burdens weighed down my spirit, and yet the passion and fervor to serve remained. There were spurts of energy that would bubble up inside of me and come out in the form of a huge smile for someone that I was called to serve. Someone who needed that smile. The smile that I didn't have to give but that God nevertheless supplied me with for both my residents' sakes and my own. As Hebrews 13:21 says, "May he equip you with all you need for doing his will. *May he produce in you*, through the power of Jesus Christ, every good thing that is pleasing to him. All glory to him forever and ever! Amen" (NLT). The pressure is not on me to have strength in and of myself. I can call on the Lord and trust that He will help me to do His will as long as I have faith. This is something that I must emphasize: there was this supernatural energy that remained within me during the duration of every work shift. This energy showed itself to be very much alive through my job. The Lord's strength and the bonds that I had with my residents successfully triumphed over the personal battles that I was facing. In the crux of my deepest struggles with anxiety, I had a note on my mirror that read: "Take the very thing I'm needing and give it to someone else." This perspective will be applicable for the rest of my life.

It is so interesting to see the difference that my mindset makes for the quality of my life, and how those around me pick up on the consequences of that mindset. People can either suffer from my negative perspective or benefit from my positive one. It has been essential for me to understand that I have the choice every day, and that God gives me the powerful ability to "take captive every thought to make it obedient to Christ" (2 Corinthians 10:5, NIV). I have a mighty power at work within me that I can tap into, or I can ignore it and do a great disservice to both myself and the company that I keep.

On a daily basis, I witnessed individuals come to work with a look of dread on their faces as they drug their feet or wore a countenance of pure exhaustion. I would see their greatest energy derive from gossiping about their coworkers rather than rejoicing in the relationships that they had the potential to create. One day, my other executive director, Tracy Martin, shared a message during a meeting at work that was quite profound: "The amount of time that people spend being negative or talking about someone else is the time that is spent consequently neglecting the residents." She said that we could have fun, work as a unit, and leave the job laughing if we all stayed positive. I learned that positive energy attracts the crowd that I want to keep and gives me the strength to persist and do the right thing in the face of adversity. No matter their age and ailments, the elderly are attuned to who is trustworthy and who is not.

Oftentimes, I believe that people do not understand the vitality that servitude brings to the human heart. It is a gift that keeps on giving. Even if one is tired, they can get more energized, rather than more exhausted, from going the extra mile for another individual. I have learned that my perspective shapes my entire life, and when I choose to do good whenever there is the opportunity (Galatians 6:10), the result is that my own heart is uplifted. When I humble myself, the Lord exalts me (James 4:10). I must understand that the good I do is not dependent on how I feel or who I direct it towards, but the *spirit* in which I exercise servitude.

In which you can ask yourself:

1. What does gossip take you away from in your position as a caregiver? What are you forsaking when you engage in it?

2. Where does your energy come from day-to-day?

3. When are you most tempted to be selfish in your position as a caregiver, and what are some examples of what selfishness would look like? Does accessibility to your phone affect the kind of attention and care you are giving to those around you?

4. What are the *intentions* that your actions are rooted in?

Chapter Seven:

Paternalism

Dear Reader,

As caregivers, I hope that we can all understand that servitude never equals superiority. Trying to change anyone is a form of control that always ends in exhaustion and misery. Respect is a supreme form of charity. I hope that amidst the many job responsibilities and the haste of day-to-day life, you remember to listen for the voices beneath the noise. I hope that you get to know those within your care and prompt yourself to understand their personal needs, identifying them as human beings rather than objects. I hope that you never view them as children that merely need to be *taught*.

(Scribble 1) Uninhibited Freedom

Perhaps one of the most radical acts of love in this finite life is to *let* somebody be who they are. To allow them the space to blossom and grow, even when they are rooted between a mere crack in the sidewalk. No individual can change another, and an effort to do so can often be established in control and result in misery. Every person has the opportunity to draw from the well of free will that the Creator has given them. I cannot draw for another; that is an act between an individual and the Lord. While my job has never been to mold others to my image, I can surely watch the beauty of their existence unfold in the image of the Father. When they sprout, they can look back and see me with open arms of love. To accept someone *as they are* is to humble myself with the realization that I am mere dust with no reason for pride. I am given worth by the sheer grace of the Father. As scripture states, "For he knows how we are formed, he remembers that we are but dust. The life of mortals is like grass, they flourish like a flower of the field; the wind blows over it and it is gone, and its place remembers it no more" (Psalm 103: 14–16, NIV). If I am in no position to boast – and none of us are – then I am certainly not in the state to alter another's character. For so long, I thought that I knew what was best for those I cared about. I began to put two-and-two together when I realized that my own viewpoints were constantly changing. Turns out, I am a work-in-progress myself. As James M. Barrie, the creator of Peter Pan, once said: "Life is a long lesson in humility." I am only a leader when I am open to being led. To surrender control and welcome different opinions with curiosity rather than criticism is a form of meekness, humility, and love.

The gift of human companionship is to be an example, to love, to pray for, and to help others when the circumstances present themselves. It is to nourish another's body as my own and to be slow to take offense. It is to give advice out of charity, discernment, and wisdom. It is to be quick to listen, slow to speak, and slow to become angry. One day I wrote this in my journal: "Do I want to be a "good" human being? Put down everything and be an active listener (show value and care)."

Within my facility, we had home-health workers that provided extra care for a portion of our residents. One day, I got to talking to one of these workers that regularly assisted a woman named Lila. She gave me a beautiful piece of advice that I believe opens up the heart to benevolence, empathy, and compassion for others. Every morning, Lila liked to get ready in her bathroom, shave, brush her teeth, and pamper herself for the day. This often led to her missing breakfast and lunch and having to get room service delivered to her apartment. Lila's worker told me that she could either get frustrated about this or let Lila do it. She said that there is very little freedom that the elderly still have. Therefore, caregivers may as well let them have some control over their lives and not get worked up over what one may consider "inconveniences." The most profound statement that she shared, however, is as follows: "I am not here to change her, I am here to help her."

So often, the elderly are treated as if they are children that need to be trained up in the way that they should go. It is easy to adopt this paternalistic mindset in a job where someone is assisting another. However, the decency of honoring another's individuality, personhood, and what is left of their independence applies here just as much as it would for a younger adult. In fact, it would do us all well to respect our elders and regard them as the beacons of wisdom that they are. I knew that my residents had built up a life for themselves for the past seventy to ninety years, and it was not my duty to begin dismantling their buildings. I was to inspire them, be inspired *by them*, show them compassion, and learn from their stories.

(Scribble 2) Soft Voices, Unheard

They are the soft voices that are often unheard, yet should be the first ones that we are listening to. Blessed is the person who humbles himself enough to tilt his ear toward the silent cry beneath the noise. Blessed is the person who draws near to the broken-hearted and those contrite in spirit, as the Lord does (Psalm 34:18). Blessed is the person who serves the least of these, for it is then that they serve Jesus Himself (Matthew 25:40).

It is when I hearken to the voices of those around me that I am able to serve them well. It is when I dig deeper into the meaning behind an expression, the thought behind a phrase, and the possibility of a hidden need that I demonstrate genuine care for the elderly.

As Wallace Reynolds expressed, there has to be a *respect* for elders when one is working in geriatrics. Just because I was *taking care of* the elderly did not mean that I *ever* had a reason to count them as subservient to myself. I observed how disrespect is linked to neglect in many ways, and this applies to all relationships in one's life. In order to hold myself to a much higher standard of consideration for my fellow man, *my elders included*, I was to regard every person around me as God's creation.

The very act of caregiving was the agreement to enter into self-denial; it was to forget about much of what I "deserved" and to replace it with the recognition that I had, in actuality, earned nothing. Everything good that I had and continue to have is from above (James 1:17). Even my comfort from the Lord can be used to comfort others in return. As 2 Corinthians 1:4 says, "Who comforteth us in all our tribulation, that we may be able to comfort them which are in any trouble, by the comfort wherewith we ourselves are comforted of God" (KJV). Caregiving was to put my neighbor *before* myself, oftentimes at the expense of my own wants and desires. If the job did not include any traces of sacrifice, then, dare I say, it would not have been genuine. To sacrifice oneself for another is the greatest act of love. Unfortunately, because of the fallen nature of humans, even our best acts are tainted with insincerity, sin, and self-gratification. It is something that I found I must *continuously* work on to overcome. A beautiful remedy for this has been delving into scriptures like 1 Corinthians 13 and Colossians 3, writing them out, and choosing to believe them for myself. I learned that spiritual growth will be a life-long devotion.

In anything that I do, I believe it to be vitally important that I keep first things first from the very beginning. My actions must be preceded by foundational goals if I intend on abiding by my values when things get rough. When a caregiver loses sight of the *opportunity* to connect with others in a profound way, they lose sight of their purpose. Therefore, the quality of their work begins to decline. I had to regularly re-focus to remind myself of the person that I wanted to be and the difference that I wanted to make. This was not just for the sake of the job, but in the grand scheme of my life. The human brain is naturally self-centered, so service is not something that comes easily to individuals. It is an armor that has to be put on each morning when I wake up and enter into a new day. Some days, my armor falls off before nighttime arrives, and other times it is hanging off of my shoulder. No matter what, I ask for forgiveness and start again.

As Mr. Reynolds once told me, it is important to focus on the residents first and look out for their needs, and everything else seems to fall into place. My job is to not turn a deaf ear to those that I am called to serve. I am not to let my *wants* get in the way of the *needs* of those around me.

An important lesson that I came to understand in the field of geriatrics is that the elderly still possess the same traits as the youth. The only difference is that their habits have been further impressed into their character through years of practice. When I looked at my residents as works in progress rather than completed pieces, I began to understand the normalcy of imperfections in their personalities. Insecurities, temper tantrums, and a lack of knowledge remain even in old age. Sometimes the elderly – especially those living with memory loss – do not even realize *what* daily practices are beneficial for their well-being. This occurs often, and I believe it to be the caregivers' job to prompt those that they are caring for to do things that they know to be good for them. Of course, it is also important to examine which activities are fitting for each person's abilities. For example, my resident, Grace, was living with moderate dementia and would sometimes say no to the things she wanted to say yes to and vice versa. She was someone who spent most of her day in her wheelchair in the community room with nothing to do except eat cookies, drink coffee, and wait for someone to come in the front doors. Therefore, I knew it would be great for her health to have a change of scenery. Instead of *asking* if she wanted to go for a stroll outside, I would just take her during my extra time throughout my shift or after I got off of work.

Sometimes in this field, it is in the residents' best interest not to *ask* them what they want to do, but just to plan for an activity and have them engage in it. Often, they may not be fully aware of what is taking place, but they will notice the positive effects on their body in hindsight. For instance, after I took Grace for a stroll one afternoon, I heard her say to herself, "That was nice. She took me out on the little merry-go-round. And it just felt so good to be out there."

Another example of this is Mr. Thomas, who also had memory loss and would constantly tell the story of a time when he would play dominoes with the other residents. He did not remember that some of his friends in the facility had moved away and others had passed. However, he *was able* to look back fondly on a time when he felt a great sense of community and purpose. Now, my job was to use these context clues of his *past* needs in order to formulate a way in which he would be able to reconnect with himself in the *present*. While there were no longer other dominoes players in the community, I also recognized that Thomas would ask about the newspaper nearly every day. I asked him if he wanted to play Bingo, which was an activity that other people in our community engaged in. To this recommendation, he replied with a laugh and told me that Bingo was a game that requires no thought. With that information, I now understood that he enjoyed activities that picked his brain and offered intellectual engagement. Sudoku, puzzles, and magazines came to mind, all of which proved to be topics of interest to Thomas!

In order to meet my residents' personal needs – yet again – I truly had to make the effort to *get to know* those that I cared for. Just as my best friends know what is good for me when I am struggling, I had some remedies up my sleeve for when my residents were going through dark seasons of life.

In which you can ask yourself:

1. What do you know about the person within your care that you can utilize to make their life more joyful? What are they saying "no" to when they mean to say "yes"?

2. How can you incorporate the past of the person within your care into their present reality? How creative can you get?

3. Would you help your best friend in a dark season of their life? How can you see your elders through that same lens and help/serve them?

Chapter Eight:

Inspiration

Dear Reader,

I hope that this chapter inspires you with the understanding that those we are called to bless are equally as much of a blessing to *us*. There are wonderful lessons to be learned from the hearts and personalities of the people within one's care. Living in a time and society where we can adopt the mindset that the world owes us something, I hope that we remember to stay humble and kind. When we realize that we truly deserve nothing, every little thing becomes a sweet gift. It takes a beautiful person to see beauty in another. May you remember that what you behold with your eyes is a reflection of your own soul. May we all be humbled by our own failures in the light of God's mercy and grace.

(Scribble 1) Poetry and Inspiration

The greatest inspiration that I have acquired is seeing the double-sided effect of servanthood in those that I have cared for. In hindsight, my residents have served my life just as much as I have served theirs, if not more. It is beautiful to be able to look back on my life and see the handprints of God and His miraculous touch through the ones that I *appeared* to be assisting. I have come to know that I am a mere creation serving another, and anything good that takes place in that servanthood is credited to the Creator. Nothing good comes to me that has not been given from above, and my residents have been a showcase of His goodness in the day-to-day aspects of life.

My residents have shown me that there is the opportunity to serve wherever we are, no matter the age or the limitation to one's condition. As long as there is breath in my lungs, there is a purpose in that very breath. While society tells me to do what makes me happy, my soul longs for meaning beyond a self-gratifying life.

Phillip and Tammy were a married couple that lived in our assisted living center. They were former missionaries with beautiful hearts and an apartment that housed their dog, Poppy. Through sickness and health, falls and setbacks, they did not allow their circumstances to hinder their duty to serve the ones around them. Every week, Phillip would come up with a topic and host a Bible study for the other residents at the facility. More than once, I found Tammy sitting on the couch in their apartment with a Bible in her lap.

Gladys and Hamilton were another pair of companions, who had both lost their spouses and cleaved to each other in a beautiful friendship. Wherever Gladys was, it was assumed that Hamilton would be there and vice versa; the two were inseparable. Gladys grew up in a family of five sisters where her mother taught them to be dedicated to the Lord and loving others, while her father taught them to drink their coffee black. Hamilton was a former engineer who had many stories to tell about things he had accomplished and places he had traveled for work. Now, the couple spent most of their days soaking in the sunshine on the front porch or in the sun room with the radio playing beside them. One day, I even caught sight of them dancing together through the front window. They would often meet me with a greeting when I came in for my shift and wave at me when it was my time to go home. It was a frequent occurrence for Gladys to look at me and say, "Thank you for all that you do," with a smile. One day, when I was working the front desk during the COVID-19 pandemic, I found myself having two extra sets of helping hands from these extraordinary individuals. They helped me lug in boxes from the mail without being asked or expected to do such a kind deed. I overheard Gladys say to her partner in well-doing, "Come on, Hamilton, we have some work to do." In another instance, she told him, "If you see somebody who needs some help, go out and help 'em." Even with the onset of memory loss, who Gladys was at her core remained the motivating factor for her actions. Gladys had scripture written on her heart, Ephesians 5:15–16 coming to mind with her benevolent words: "Look carefully then how you walk, not as unwise but as wise, making the best use of the time, because the days are evil" (ESV).

It is beautiful to see that who someone is in their spirit long outlives who they are in their flesh. I am quite convinced that my memory will always preserve a spot for sweet Delilah Poe: a lady I came to know and love when I first started my job in geriatric care. She was the cutest little woman in the memory care unit, petite in stature yet slightly plump in width. She was known for her requests for a snack multiple times a day, and would usually settle down with a bowl of Raisin Bran. Her pointy-toed shoes, much like her, were worn out with age but full of character. Although often riddled with anxiety, shaking legs, and memory loss, Delilah Poe had the most golden heart of anyone I had ever met. She was always worried about everyone else. When you asked her how she was doing, she would often respond with, "And how are *you* doing, honey?" in the most dainty and loving voice. If you did anything kind for her, she would treat you like an angel. However, *she* was, in fact, the angel; I truly believe that it takes a beautiful person to notice beauty in others. Delilah Poe was an avid lover of back scratches and foot massages. She could often be found carrying around a devotional or scouring the bookshelf in the memory care unit. Her Bible could be found in her room, and her faith radiated from her personality. She truly was a city set on a hill and a light in the world; a light that still sticks with me to this day.

My resident, Emily, often encouraged me in my Christianity. She would point it out when she witnessed me walking in Jesus' footsteps. Even at the age of ninety-two, she had a quote that she tried to read every day that shaped her perspective on how she was to treat others. Her and I would have deep conversations about faith over her nightly foot massages. During election season, she told me that she prayed to the Lord, "Create in me a clean heart, O' God, and renew a right spirit within me." Afterwards, she said, "And then I felt better about Trump again." A funny statement albeit a beautiful one. How often we allow our hearts to be hardened toward others, projecting our fears and rejections onto them. As Emily showcased that night, God wants to do something beautiful in our souls *when* they are soft and teachable, and dwelling on our frustrations prevents that from happening. Caregiving is no exception to this opportunity for character growth, and may even be one of the primary examples of it. Emily once paraphrased a beautiful line from Elisabeth Kubler-Ross: "People are like stained glass windows. They sparkle and shine when all is sunny and bright, but their true beauty is only seen when there is a light from within." One Sunday, Emily caught me in the dining hall and asked me to come see her later that evening. It turns out that she had written down a sermon from that morning to share with me. This sermon was one that spoke to my life situation at the time. Two profound quotes from the message are as follows: 1) "If you try sitting on two chairs, you end up falling on the floor. Choose one." 2) "When you're chasing two rabbits, you won't catch either one." I was hoping that she would allow me to keep that piece of paper so that I could cherish it my whole life . . . and she did. She complained that the handwriting was messy. "But it's *your* handwriting," I said. That's all that mattered.

Sometimes, when I would walk with Lila to and from the bathroom in her apartment, she would sing this song: "Good morning, Lord! It's a beautiful day! / Good morning, Lord! I'm going your way! / Open my eyes, that I may see, someone who needs a friend like me. / I know that I will surely be loving, caring, always sharing. / Good morning, Lord! I'm going your way!" After working with Lila for two years, I knew the song by heart. She inspired a tenderness within me, and I believe that that's exactly what she *meant* to do when she sang the melody alongside her caregivers. The last day I saw her, I was told that she was not much longer for this world. I was able to share a few final moments with her. "Lila, it's Kayla. Lila, it's Kayla," I would say, and I would get a move of her hand in response. That was enough, and I didn't realize the significance of that until she was gone. She passed away about thirty minutes later. Sometimes, we don't realize the weight of someone's presence until they are no longer tangible. Lila had that sort of presence, and I had that sort of realization when she was no longer around.

Lenora was an extremely talented resident of mine. I remember when her and her husband, Frederick, had just moved into the facility. She had me stack her book shelves with a plethora of insightful publications. As a former RN and artist, she had an abundance of medical guides, followed by books filled with art and various patterns for inspiration. As I got to work helping her make the new apartment feel like home, she told me about her life. When I asked her how she knew her husband was the one, she said: "He liked my legs, and I liked his voice." Lenora and Frederick enjoyed bird-watching in their younger years and had a beautiful home in Rockville, Maryland. Her and her husband bubbled over with excitement to show me the blanket that Lenora had been working on. The mere undertaking of such a lofty project was both inspirational and phenomenal. As she spread the huge cover across her bed for me to view, I was moved to amazement. The intricate detail was a display of her and Frederick's old backyard. Every stitch was done with complexity in mind: the blue path with tiny yellow flowers, the various animals scattered throughout the yard, a blue squirrel with a fluffy tail, a brick gate, and gigantic trees. She had also painted a picture based off of that same backyard and personalized it so that it captured the memories that her and Frederick shared. There was the stray cat that would hide in the bushes, the black snake that they would often see, a fox, and a variety of birds. That home was a sanctuary to them; a place to look back on in remembrance and appreciation. Lenora's art pieces were a way to keep those memories alive and present *wherever* she was.

I left their room so inspired and so filled with the idea that I can pursue what I love and be a blessing to others through my passions. Rather than finding my worth in people, I can find joy in what I can contribute to them through the creativity that I have been given. In fact, it was such a heartening experience that Lenora remarked, "Wow. I'm gonna call you Miss Wow" because of how many times I said the word during our time together!

And those books that I stacked on her shelves? Lenora's son had refused to help her, telling her to throw all of them away. As Lenora told *me* and as I encourage *you*, my reader, "Don't do that to your parents (or those within your care). Let them keep their stuff. It's what they have."

(Scribble 2) Passions are Cultivated

When I interviewed Wallace Reynolds, he told me that someone does not do geriatric work until they have experienced being around the elderly. This sounds simple but proved to be true, as I did not fall in love with the geriatric population until I immersed myself in my job as a caregiver. In fact, Mr. Reynolds started out by spending time with his grand-dad, and then went on to become the executive director of an entire assisted living building. People without a passion do not usually make it in this kind of work for the long-haul. However, I realized that individuals often don't recognize the area and depth of their interests until they explore the opportunities around them. When I began university, I decided to pursue a degree in English. While I will always be an avid writer, for much of my life I was deprived of the knowledge that I also find fulfillment in one-on-one care. I began to understand that the most valuable writings are cultivated through life experiences and nurtured relationships, and I saw this first-hand through my job in geriatrics.

I believe that humans can fall in love with what they cater to in their lives. Like my friend, Elisabeth, said: "Passions are cultivated, not birthed." I believe that each person has God-given gifts instilled within them. However, I have come to know that it is my duty to cultivate those very gifts that I have been given into something beautiful and productive for His Kingdom. Perhaps I would not have fallen in love with the elderly like I did if I wasn't immersed in an environment in which I could cater to the passion within me. In the same way, I might have had a similar passion for children if I involved myself in a teaching position abroad with little ones hanging at my hip. With the heart for caregiving that I found in myself, it could have been cultivated in a number of ways. It is not only my job to continue nurturing it so that it demonstrates God's love and glory *wherever* I go, but to meet the needs that I see in the world with *any* gifts that I have been given. Underneath the rumble of all the other tumultuous beckonings in the world, geriatric care is a need that is desperately yearning to be vocalized and met in our society today. As scripture says, "As we have therefore opportunity, let us do good unto all *men*, especially unto them who are of the household of faith" (Galatians 6:10, KJV).

One time, Elisabeth and I spent part of an evening with one of my ninety-five year-old residents, Ollie. After expressing to us that he thought the world had gone to shambles, he said, "Nobody's satisfied with anything anymore." He made a good point, as much of society has been brainwashed by greed and lack of contentment. As Mr. Reynolds told me, the older generation does not have the expectations that the younger generations have. They are content with merely having a good place to stay and being cared for, while the generations to come are individuals that never feel as if they have *enough*. Our world has been so consumed by sin and self-gratification that it is going to require a lot of contemplation, prayer, and life changes to get out of the twisted assumption that any of us deserve anything. One of the beautiful qualities about my residents was their gratitude. My job as a caregiver taught me that life is not to be lived in self-focus, and that a heart that is passionate about servanthood is one in which must be cultivated. I am to be satisfied with what I have and to use what I've been given to give to others.

I have come to the conclusion that we need people in this world who are willing to have adaptable lives for the sake of others. For a long while, I had a quote on my mirror that read something to the effect of, "To be the kind of person who makes plans but doesn't get upset when those plans change." I have learned that flexibility is one of the greatest acts of selflessness. Indeed, Jesus stopped in the middle of His journey to confront the woman who touched his garment. He acted in spite of the pressure of the engulfing crowd and His disciples urging Him to keep going. He was not too busy to be flexible for His fellow man, for He knew of the important things in life.

The act of caring does not cease when a work-shift is over. It is not limited by time, personal wants, or plans. It does not prioritize material things over the affirmation of someone else's worth. Passions are cultivated by the kind of service they render; what is left of my passions when my physical presence no longer graces this earth is what is important to me. It is not the gift in and of itself that is important. It is the *soul* of the gift; the invisible impression that the gift leaves behind that no one can take away.

You see, love beckons me to look deeper. It begs me to ask what someone might have been through. It leads me to acknowledge that I never have and never will completely live in the shoes of another, no matter how much I try and empathize. I am humbled by my own brokenness and the acknowledgement that I am the creation, not the Creator. I see that there is no partiality among sinners; I am just as messy as everyone else. Therefore, just as I have been made worthy of grace, I am not in a position to measure whether or not someone else is worthy. My job was and is to give of it freely, as I have been given. Mercy is unmerited for all of us, no matter who we are or what we have done.

I come from the perspective that it is not completely true that people don't *want* to go the extra mile. In fact, I think that many have never been shown *how* to. Service may seem to be an obvious act of the will, but I have experienced how unfair that assumption can be numerous times in my life. Often, the simple act of being led by example motivates people to understand the need for change in the world. One day, my coworker that I had trained nearly a year prior stated that she had no idea that giving the residents foot massages was not a part of the job responsibilities. That was the way that I had shown her to approach caregiving, and it was something that stuck with her until she was told differently. As simple as it may sound, humans often don't feel comfortable being different until someone else leads the way and lets them know it's okay. To be a person who leads in kindness is my life goal. Sometimes, kindness puts people in awkward positions because it is not expected in our individualistic culture, but it is *always* worth a shot. As someone who has always been naturally shy, I have learned that awkwardness is a harmless version of vulnerability that every individual who pursues service will encounter. The best part is that most people who feel awkward about being the recipients of such service are more stunned, awed, and humbled than deterred. They are moved that such benevolence can occur in this harsh world. I like to say that going the extra mile is two times as difficult and four times as rewarding. Being joyfully blessed by being a blessing should never be the end goal, but it can most certainly be the result.

In which you can ask yourself:

1. In what ways can you let the person within your care inspire *you*?

2. What "stuff" do the people within your care want to keep? (This "stuff" can either be tangible or a part of their inner self that you can help protect as their caregiver.)

Chapter Nine:

COVID-19

Dear Reader,

It doesn't take a pandemic to realize that there is a shortage of love throughout our world today. There are compromises to be made in the face of differences. There is also a grave need for inwardness in the face of overexertion and cultural busyness. The oppression of COVID-19 has merely been a large awakening to the oppressions that humans face day-to-day. It has also been an invitation to learn how individuals can face opposition with the strength of the Lord.

(Scribble 1) The Oppression of COVID-19

The spring and summer of 2020 proved to be an awakening time for me in my pursuit of geriatric care. The COVID-19 pandemic brought with it new challenges for my facility to face head-on. Although added responsibilities were heaped onto the staff, the residents could not escape from the reality of the virus like we could. I was able to leave for home at the end of my shifts, but home quickly became a prison for some of my residents.

The pandemic brought to light aspects of assisted living that were essential to the quality of life of those within my care. Because of the virus, every time one of my residents had to leave the facility for any medical appointments, they had to be quarantined for fourteen days following their return. This added the component of isolation on top of the sacrifices that the elderly *already* have to make in regards to their independence day-to-day. It made me realize how much they look forward to simple interactions with their peers, such as going to the dining hall three times a day for their meals. Sometimes, food is about the only thing that the elderly can muster up the strength to get out of their rooms for. With COVID-19, one of my residents had to get room service for two weeks. I asked her about this experience afterwards, and she informed me that her meals were cold by the time they arrived to her room. Sadly, this is one of the aspects of a care-facility that residents have to accept when they make the trade-off for the dining hall. Even if the room service trays are to be delivered as soon as they come out of the kitchen, there is additional time added to distribute the trays to the various rooms and individual halls. Other contributing factors to this delay include pagers going off, understaffing, and other job responsibilities begging the caregivers for attention.

Lila looked forward to getting dressed up every day, as well as having her personal caregiver take her into town to interact with the community. Due to COVID-19, this was no longer possible. An essential part of her character was stripped away. The hours she slept grew longer, and the amount of time it took for her to get dressed every day extended. She was an integral part of the community center in her younger years and was used to being very active in the town. Lila was an ambitious soul with an intelligent and creative mind. It meant the world to her to visit with others, receive a hand-written note, or share her beautiful love story and letters that her and her husband exchanged in their youth. Lila could be found donning bright red lipstick, painted nails, eyeshadow, and blush. As long as she had breath in her lungs, she had motivation to live rather than merely survive.

Cicely was another one of my residents that was impacted by COVID-19. She was an eighty-five year-old woman that was full of life and would naturally put others before herself. She used to visit a one-hundred year-old in the memory care unit from time to time and would bring her little brown chihuahua, Lilly, along to visit. The other residents absolutely LOVED Lilly, and she easily became a sort of therapy dog to lift their spirits with her sweet nature and petite size. Cicely would play Bingo in the activity room while Lilly rested on top of her walker. She would also take the tiny dog for walks around the building. Of course, she would make sure to stop by the community couch on the way inside to let her jump up and visit with the residents. The two were inseparable. She would often refer to the little dog as "pumpkin," which was a perfect portrayal of Cicely's sweet heart. One time, I walked into Cicely's room, and she was making homemade smores with chocolate graham crackers, Nutella, peanut butter, and marshmallows. She told me that she was "experimenting." Apparently, I was destined to experiment with her. It was during this visit that I could easily see myself becoming best friends with this woman. There we were: sitting side by side on her couch, eating our homemade smores, with Lilly licking any extra peanut butter off of our fingers.

One day, Cicely was begrudgingly transported to the hospital after having dizziness and chest pain. However, because of the required quarantine, she knew that leaving the facility would mean that she couldn't walk her dog when she returned. On top of that, fourteen days trapped inside of a room for someone that is fairly active left her feeling stir crazy. Fortunately, Lilly and I became great pals and sleeping buddies as I took her for visits to my apartment while Cicely was unable to care for her.

Perhaps the most heartbreaking of all was the fact that the residents were not allowed to have visitors. My resident, June, and her husband had been married for fifty-six years. She had become wheelchair bound, required hand-feedings, and was not very responsive. It was evident to me that the last phase of her life was crucial for her husband to be a part of, and this virus stripped away some of those precious moments. She passed away in August of 2020, a few months after the virus began. When my resident, Frank, came down with COVID-19 and was transported to another facility, I called to inquire about visiting him. I was told that he was in the "COVID unit," and that visitors were not allowed in that area. When the virus broke out in our memory care unit, my resident, Elsy, tested negative but was still required to quarantine. One day, when she was sitting in her wheelchair in her room, I asked her how she was feeling. She responded, "Abandoned. I need my friends." She was used to being around other people her age, and all of her peers were sick, had passed away, were out of the facility, or were stuck in their apartments.

After Christmas, when COVID-19 was still running rampant in the world, I went to Charlotte's room to deliver some sweets. I found this note on her door for all to see: "I am here. Please wake me up. I want to see you." After knocking on her door, I was met with eyes that were red and watery: allergies mixed with sad tears. Our interaction was filled with Charlotte telling me that it was the first Christmas she had ever spent alone. We hugged, she cried, and her spirits were uplifted by the sweets. She told me that I had come at just the right time, and I told her that it was the divine alignment of the Lord. Charlotte's sensitive soul did not respond well to isolation. She expressed her loneliness to me more than once throughout the pandemic, and even wondered aloud if being stuck in her room was a form of punishment.

One of my residents by the name of Ivy thrived the most when she was outside. She was an avid nature lover with a heart for God's creation. You could often see her standing outside, peering ahead in wonder. The sound of birds was music to her ears, and her ninety + year-old body was still well-equipped for physical exercise. Hattie, who had progressively become walking buddies with Ivy, was a humorous woman who would stroll around with her walker before bed in order to alleviate anxiety fueled by her memory loss. During COVID-19, it made it more difficult to accommodate both of these women, as the doors were locked by six p.m. every night. On multiple occasions, Hattie would ask if she could walk outside after dinner, or Ivy would sigh in exasperation at the fact that her time outdoors was limited by the virus. Going outside meant taking the risk of being locked out, as evening shifts are busy and it is impossible for caregivers to watch everyone at once. This added another layer of frustration and confusion to the residents' weary minds. This was the perfect opportunity to go the extra mile and walk with them after work with a rock or pillow propping the door open. Although the situation wasn't ideal, compromises are often necessary in times of change.

Thanks to our wonderful program director, Lana Smith, who had been working at the facility for sixteen years, her heart of compassion created a way for the elderly to FaceTime their families. I could see how emotional, uplifting, and stimulating this was to the minds of my residents. Even Mrs. Smith was moved by one-hundred year-old resident, Isaac, FaceTiming with his son from his bed-bound state. Isaac's age had led to his bodily decline, and he relied completely on staff for his personal hygiene and food delivery services. Nonetheless, he nearly always had such a sweet, humorous demeanor and a positive outlook on life! It was heartwarming to see his son visit nearly every day after the COVID-19 limitations were reduced. Similarly, Mrs. Smith gave Gladys the opportunity to FaceTime with her family. I considered this to be such a precious gift, as Gladys' memory was progressively deteriorating. It quickly dawned on me that the virus didn't wait for anyone. Therefore, these were crucial moments that Gladys was able to share with her loved ones.

One of my elderly friends experienced the loss of her husband and had to live alone throughout the extent of the virus. In response to this, she expressed to me the following simple and heartbreaking truth: "I'm not used to being by myself. I had two sisters and a mommy and daddy when I came into the world."

(Scribble 2) Patience Running Thin

As COVID-19 began to subtly affect our workers at the facility, the true test of character within me began to emerge. One's patience is tried when tiredness sinks in and expectations from others seem unfairly demanding. As multiple caregivers came down with the virus, understaffing and overworking permeated our building. Some of my coworkers were stuck working sixteen + hour shifts. We only had two overnight caregivers remaining, so they were stretched to the limit. People that worked overnight began their duties at ten p.m. and finished at six in the morning. This was not a first choice for many caregivers and therefore resulted in a shortage of help. One of the girls was merely eighteen years old and was working the night shift so frequently that she chose to move into one of the empty apartments. Another worker was already going through a very difficult season of life and became evidently burnt out on everything. Her spirit was downcast, and her motivation to keep going was nearly lost altogether. More than once, she told me that she felt like she was going to go crazy, and I could tell by the exhaustion on her face that she was over-extending.

The staff were scattered all over the place. People were working different shifts than usual; the cleaning ladies could even be found working the front desk! One day, I was scheduled for the assisted living section of the building and got moved to the memory care unit because someone had to leave early. This left my coworker in assisted living to do both her job and mine by *herself*. Therefore, there was no time to shower the residents that were scheduled that day. In other words, there was no room for anyone to take off work without someone else getting the short end of the stick.

This was during a summer in my life where I was packing up to move, writing this book, and working immensely more than I had during the school year. I was beginning to get worn down during a time when there was no room to be worn. College tuition for the spring semester was approaching, new rent payments would need to be met, and I had a loan to pay off and other expenses to look forward to. On top of this, my dad had an upcoming surgery for prostate cancer, and my mom had also been given a diagnosis. My job was not to heap more burdens onto my parents but to alleviate the ones that they had as much as I could. Even *without* the difficulties that COVID-19 had brought along, taking off of work wouldn't have been an intelligent choice . . . or a considerate one.

The more I was contacted to pick up different shifts, the more used I began to feel. It threatened to affect my patience with other workers as well as with the residents. I began to grow more hasty in my job duties and less willing to do extra chores. My back began to hurt after lifting people, and this triggered concern about long-term back issues. During this time just as much as any, the residents needed my patience and joyful spirit. Being aware of my own irritation and where it was coming from was crucial for me. There were three things that I knew I needed: more rest, more Bible study, and a frequent change of scenery. Instead of exercising after work one evening, I read 1 Corinthians 13 and called it a night. The following morning, I got up and read Colossians 3: "Clothe yourselves as God's own chosen ones (His own picked representatives), [who are] purified and holy and well-beloved [by God Himself, by putting on behavior marked by kind feeling, a lowly opinion of yourselves, *gentle ways*, [and] *patience, which is tireless and long-suffering, and has the power to endure whatever comes, with good temper]*" (AMP).

It is verses such as this one that allow me to refocus throughout my life when I begin to feel discombobulated. I am reminded of my purpose on this earth to represent the Lord well alongside the ways in which I am called to do just that. Patience endures long and is a form of love, and gentleness is exceedingly tender in His sight.

Additionally, there was a particular moment during this hectic time that the Lord used fellowship with one of my best friends, Maddi, to restore my energy when I was feeling run-down. We walked and jogged around my neighborhood, chit-chatted, let her German shepherd wet his feet in the ditch, and went on a Sonic-run for iced Big Red. This simple pleasure was enough to give me an enthusiasm for life once again and ready me for my shift at work later that day. Of course, by the time the day was over I felt like I needed another boost, but it was a great reminder to cling to the little blessings for longer. It also humbled me with the reality that I am an imperfect human being. You, my dear reader, are also an imperfect human being. You can only give of love freely when you freely receive it. You can only live according to your values when you take a moment to stop and ask yourself *what* exactly those values *are*. Allow your own bucket to be filled, and then share that bucket with those you are called to love!

In which you can ask yourself:

1. What sacrifices do the elderly have to make on a day-to-day basis in regards to their independence?

2. What memories can you share with the ones within your care? Can you take a moment to sit on the couch with them and bond over some homemade smores?

3. What do *you* need in order to remain strengthened for the sake of those within your care? Can you come up with a list of things that you can do to refuel daily?

4. How can you show yourself grace as an imperfect human being and, therefore, as an imperfect caregiver?

Chapter Ten:

Loving Those with Memory Loss

Dear Reader,

My hope is that this chapter will provide some insight into the sweet approach that those with memory loss respond best to. May you look at the actions of others through a lens that always believes the best. Please remember that difficult responses from those within your care could be an indication of a deeper need.

(Scribble 1) The Confused Mind Still Recognizes Love

"Above all, love each other deeply, because love covers over a multitude of sins" (1 Peter 4:8, NIV)

Even in the absence of memory and adequate bodily function, I am a believer that the soul is still able to recognize love. I believe it because I have seen it firsthand and have witnessed the healing properties of charity to a broken spirit.

I have also seen love be withdrawn, as if it is a right to be taken away as soon as an individual's mind starts to grow weak. It is easy to adopt the attitude of superiority when a person begins to lose an aspect of their body that is so essential to their humanity: their brain. Respect can be replaced with the perspective that those living with Alzheimer's and dementia are "out of their minds" or – as I have heard more than one person say – "crazy."

Yet, I observed a distinct difference when a resident living with memory loss was talked to with a voice of tenderness rather than a voice of authority. It was beautiful to see the responses that my residents had to a spirit of kindness. No matter how damaged the mind may be, there is something lovely about the fact that one spirit still recognizes good in the spirit of another. There is something that surpasses the tangible, physical, and visible well-being of an individual and crosses over into the invisible.

One time, I watched and listened to a coworker treat one of my residents, Grace, like a little girl. Grace may have been living with the onset of dementia, but she was still aware of her environment and emotions. In fact, she was easily one of the silliest personalities in our facility. This fellow worker of mine looked at Grace's deficits and approached her with a position of authority. I heard her commanding Grace with directives such as, "Brush your teeth," as well as ordering her to stay in her wheelchair in the hallway while she attended to another resident. The tone of voice utilized was crucial, as it resembled that of a parent reprimanding a child.

One time in particular, my coworker left Grace in the hallway, and she began to scream, "Help, help!" As my coworker came toward her, she said, "Grace, I *told you* I'm coming." Grace was convinced in her mind that she was going to take a trip "downtown," to which the caregiver responded, "You're *not* going downtown" and wheeled her to her room against her will. Later on, I went to check on Grace after she was put to bed and found her lying there *so* upset. As I stroked her hair, she expressed her frustration to me. She told me that "that woman" is just "*mean*," has a "*mean streak*," that she dragged her in there, and that she would never let her into her home. Grace felt the need to prove her individuality and repeatedly said, "I have a *good* reputation!" She told me that she could just get her bags and leave. The sad reality was that Grace was already deprived of this aspect of her independence and felt as if the caregiver had stripped her of even more freedom.

In the midst of her frustration, Grace told me: "I'm ninety years old," as if to assert her need for receiving esteem. Our elders need to be respected. The sad part is that some people do not know how to treat their own parents and grandparents with honor, and this translates over into how they treat those they care for. I do not think that my coworker *meant* to treat Grace with dishonor. However, I *do* think that she was not shown a better way to demonstrate the tender love that Grace responded best to. She paralleled the resident's lack of mental clarity with a reason to neglect her personhood. Instead of *ordering* her to brush her teeth, Grace was a woman that responded cooperatively to her caregiver *asking* her if she'd *like* to brush her teeth. Grace was someone who was repulsed by the idea of being transferred into the shower. Therefore, to honor her wishes while also maintaining her hygiene, I would put her on the toilet and give her a sponge bath. I learned that I was present to help those who needed assistance, not to babysit or parent them.

A few days later, I walked into work, and Grace looked me straight in the face and said, "Thank you," with a matter-of-fact tone of voice. She didn't have the words – or perhaps even the memory – to express exactly what she was thankful for, but she knew in her spirit that someone was there for her during a hard time. As a dear friend and mentor of mine, Ruth Harper, once said: "People will forget what you did, but they will never forget how you made them feel."

With this being said, I learned for myself that no method is fool-proof. It was a few weeks after this observation that I was confronted with Grace's confusion in a way that I had never seen it before: directed at *me*. While another coworker and myself were clipping Grace's nails and painting them for her, her mind was convinced that we had kidnapped her and wouldn't let her see her family. It was humbling moments such as this one where I learned to empathize with the efforts of my fellow staff. Sometimes, no matter what a caregiver does, the resident is still not happy. Nevertheless, I believe that the best approach generally still stands: comfort, encourage, affirm, reassure, and speak gently. I continuously reminded Grace that we were helping her. My co-worker informed her that we were just going to finish up her nails and then we would take her back to her room. I hugged Grace and told her how pretty her nails were. After all, confronting a resident that is not happy with an unhappy response never helps anyone! No, Grace did not calm down or believe us right away, but that was okay and a part of the imperfect aspects of caregiving. Sometimes, sweetness is met with anger from the elderly, but sweetness still must remain on the caregiver's end. I came to find that the mark of a mature caregiver is the understanding that people living with memory loss have minds that are not well but souls that are worthy of respect nonetheless. They are not shells of people; as long as they have breath in them, they are deserving of honor. I learned to not take offense or be hurt by unintended insults. Instead, I was to meet them with a heart of compassion and unconditional love that didn't skew how I viewed those I cared for. 1 Corinthians 13: 4-8 applies perfectly here: "Love is patient, love is kind. It does not envy, it does not boast, it is not proud. It does not dishonor others, it is not self-seeking, it is not easily angered, it keeps no record of wrongs. Love does not delight in evil but rejoices with the truth. It always protects, always trusts, always hopes, always perseveres. Love never fails" (NIV).

(Scribble 2) Verbal Cues for the Misunderstood

As human beings, we have the ability to write songs with the souls of our hands, to traipse through flower fields with the souls of our feet, to taste with the souls of our tongues, to listen gracefully with the souls of our ears, and to see with the souls of our eyes. Sometimes, those very eyes are the ones that we can use to see *for* others. To look for beauty in the seemingly mundane and to grasp for mercy where none is deserved.

There is an added aspect of care that accompanies serving those that are living with Alzheimer's and dementia. Caregivers' senses have to be hyper-focused and engaged if they wish to adequately treat them as the human beings that they are. As Wallace

Reynolds once told me, "When a resident is acting up, it usually means there is a need that is not being met." For example, one of my memory care residents had the need to smoke when it was raining outside. Therefore, he brought his cigarette indoors, which was both prohibited and disrespectful to the other residents in the locked unit. In order to accommodate this need in a way that was friendly for everyone, Mr. Reynolds made sure that the resident was provided with an umbrella so that he could both smoke and stand outside without getting wet. While it can be argued that smoking is not as much a need as it is a desire, it is not the job of the staff to inform residents of their unhealthy habits. Rather, their choices are to be respected and honored in a community that is considered to be their *home*.

It can be so easy to fall into the trap of desensitization toward individuals who cannot express themselves like the average person can. It is as if faulty senses are equated with someone being less of a human being. I learned that I had to embrace my multidimensional self in order to tap into the needs of those living with Alzheimer's and dementia. These necessities were exhibited in the form of numerous cues; they could include anything from slurred phrases that resembled real words to body movements that were suggesting discomfort or a hidden need.

The most essential foundation for embracing this kind of service was caring deeply about the people in which I was assisting. Had I not cared, many cues would have slipped my notice. This could have potentially left the dementia resident suffering in silence. I could not allow the prioritization of job duties to take precedence over my concern for the wellbeing of those I was called to serve. When one of my dementia residents was shaking her leg, I came to know that this indicated that she was anxious. With this knowledge, I could therefore do my best to accommodate her so that she was more at ease. Similarly, there are a lot of things that happen behind closed doors at facilities in which workers or residents may not be aware of. This is not anyone's fault in specific but needs to be acknowledged and monitored for cautionary reasons. For example, one day I went to the room of a resident who managed her own pills. On that occasion in particular, she had already ingested her pain pill for the day. However, I caught her taking another tablet out of the bottle and told her that she had already taken it. She looked at her medicine organizer and said, "You're right honey, I did." It is situations like this that can contribute to "easy" mistakes as someone transitions from being an assisted living resident to a memory care resident.

As I get to know the people in my life, I naturally grow more competent at reading their emotions. The same should be the case for a caregiver/client relationship. I learned that if a caregiver is not willing to get to know their residents as they would get to know a friend or a family member, they are not interested or prepared enough for the job. Work should be approached with loving and respectful curiosity for the ones in which an individual works with and works *for*. This is rooted in the perspective that individuals are created to serve and put others before themselves without partiality for one person over another. As scripture says, "If anyone has material possessions and sees a brother or sister in need but has no pity on them, how can the love of God be in that person?" (1 John 3:17, NIV). This does not just include brothers and sisters by blood; as stated by Jesus: "For whosoever shall do the will of my Father which is in heaven, the same is my brother, and sister, and mother" (Matthew 12:50, KJV).

(Scribble 3) Unoffended by Inconsistency

Something that I have found to be of supreme importance when working with those living with Alzheimer's and dementia is the understanding that their personalities will not always be consistent. As someone who is very sensitive, I had to learn to take other people's actions with a grain of salt. Especially when it comes to those living with memory loss, I had to grasp the fact that there is often more than one reason behind why people act the way they do. People are very complex *without* a disease of the mind and extraordinarily complex *with* one.

Throughout my life, I have deeply struggled with being a people-pleaser and wanting everyone to love me. Unresolved conflicts have made me anxious, and I am inclined to hate confrontation. After talking about my love life to one of my residents that had just turned 103, she told me something that I needed to hear: "It sounds like you want a perfect life, tied in a pretty bow." Working as a caregiver, however, made me realize that each individual is so very intricate and unpredictable. The elderly are sometimes set in their ways, as they have had a lifetime to practice and solidify most of their day-to-day habits and perspectives. I learned that the concept of perpetual agreement is inconsistent with the very act of living. Maturing into an adult taught me (and continues to teach me) that I was not made to conform to anyone else's opinions or expectations of me. In fact, the only way that I can love someone properly is to detach from them and embrace the unique life that I have been given. I could not always make my residents happy, nor can I do so for my friends, family, or coworkers. Most importantly, *that is okay.* As someone who is very analytical, I tend to perceive people's emotions quite deeply based on their outward actions. This contributed to a lot of stress in my life before I learned that I am not meant to carry everyone's feelings. As a pastor once told me: I am responsible *to* people, not *for* people. My feelings are separate from the feelings of those around me. The less mindful I am about my individuality, the less I am able to think clearly enough to demonstrate *true* love and empathy.

My resident, Grace, and I were very close. I would walk into the building and demonstrate my excitement to see her with a huge wave and a hug. A big smile would grace her beautiful face, a cute little dress and a simple jacket adorning her body that was cradled in a wheelchair. Her and I would have what I liked to call "potty parties." I would lightheartedly stroll her to the restroom and try to be as upbeat as possible, as she'd normally feel bad about asking for the help she needed. She would call me her friend. In the same way, if I could have put her in my pocket and saved her for a rainy day, I would have. One day in particular, though, it was Grace's shower night, and she was extremely irritable. She was very resistant about being rolled to her room, as her dementia had convinced her that I was against her. She became so combative that I had to get my med-passer on duty to help me put her to bed. Even with us skipping her scheduled shower, Grace was physically aggressive as we changed her for bed and laid her down, continuously repeating the line, "How could you two do this?" She felt betrayed by the same girl that she had called her friend, and nothing that I said could convince her that we were there to help her. I felt slightly hurt that she thought so lowly of my character that night. However, she was back to normal the next day. Her memory loss tended to make people into her adversaries and invent stories that were not true.

Another resident, Kirk, had such a mental decline over the course of the two years that I had been working at the facility that he was transferred to the memory care unit. The events leading up to his transfer were his neglect of self-care, being found in the hallway with no pants or shirt on, a pillow over his privates, and his jeans strung over a random chair as he sat on the community couch. Giving Kirk showers once he reached the level of memory care was an unpredictable event. It involved much casual conversation, because he was someone that became very agitated at the feeling of being forced into any action. Commanding statements didn't work with him in the slightest. Even after successfully getting him in the shower one morning, he nearly sprayed me with water, called me names, and tried to run my foot over with his walker while I was getting him dressed. In another instance, I arrived to work and Kirk looked like he was nearly about to fall as he reached out for the chair in front of him. I put my hand out and barely touched his back for support, to which he reached out and punched me on the arm. His mind must have blamed my helping action as the reason for him nearly falling. He later apologized when he came back to his senses.

One of the most extreme cases that I observed while working in memory care was Penelope. She was in the advanced stages of memory loss, and her personality was characterized by frequent mood changes. It was interesting to observe that she was still extremely orderly and neat. This was a tendency that had apparently remained through the years and through the obstruction to her memory. I would find her with pieces of toilet paper folded and stacked up in huge piles on her apartment counter. She often made her own bed and could be found tidying up and taking dishes to the sink. She would also take it upon herself to move the chairs in the community room and thoroughly sweep the kitchen. You could hear her sighing as she completed such strenuous tasks, as if someone had forced her into doing the chores. It was evident to me that she had been a very structured, independent woman in her youth and sought to retain such qualities. Penelope would grab official paperwork if it was in her line of vision, read it, and sort through it as if it was her job to do so. If a caregiver attempted to take the papers from her, it made her very angry and agitated. When it was time to change her brief and clothes for the day, Penelope would often curse at my coworker and I, attempt to bite us, or hit us. Often, she would let out a blood-curdling scream when being assisted, and shower time was her archnemesis. Most intriguing, however, was that Penelope would go from being infuriated one second to smiling and chuckling with the flip of a switch. I grew to be extremely fond of that woman. She had such a humorous, clever smile when her mood permitted. She utterly perplexed me, but she taught me a little bit about the impermanence of emotions. Her attitude was fickle, and I learned to cherish the small glimpses of her sweetness throughout my shifts. Her and I would often exchange smiles that warmed my heart, and cooperation, gentleness, patience, and gratitude were approaches that worked generally well with her. One day, our memory care coordinator brought in a robotic cat as a therapy pet in the Alzheimer's and dementia unit. It was precious to see the curiosity that it peaked in Penelope; she approached it in observation, looking back at me to say, "Did you see that?" as the cat moved. She even looked at the animal in admiration and said, "He is so wonderful with those eyes." It was tender moments like these that I was blessed to witness, and ones in which I hold near and dear to my soul.

In which you can ask yourself:

1. Are you a cushion of grace for the one(s) within your care? Will they remember how you made them feel even if they forget what you did?

2. When a person within your care is acting out of character, what kind of needs could be begging for your attention? What is the individual being deprived of?

3. How can you prevent the juggling of job responsibilities from taking priority over the well-being and feelings of the person within your care?

4. In what ways can you be respectfully curious about the one(s) within your care and get to know them as you would get to know a friend?

5. In what ways can you practice patience and lightheartedness toward those within your care, especially the individuals who are living with memory loss?

Chapter Eleven:

Color, Humor, and a Light Heart

Dear Reader,

May this chapter demonstrate the importance of having a sweet approach with the elderly. I hope that it encourages you to have fun with your job and with those within your care. No, work does not have to be a drag! I hope that you can also see how both the environment and your personality impact the way those around you feel. May you always remember to have a light heart. We get out of life what we put into it!

(Scribble 1) A Pop of Color

"A merry heart doeth good like a medicine: but a broken spirit drieth the bones" (Proverbs 17:22, KJV).

One day, when I was spending time with my resident, Imogen, in the assisted living portion of the facility, she mentioned how depressing visiting the memory care unit was for her. She reflected on walking in and seeing the bassinet and the babies at the front of the locked unit. She perceived such a scene with a sense of dread and sympathy. However, Imogen mentioned something that got me thinking: she didn't believe that the Alzheimer's and dementia residents were actually *aware* of how chilling the environment seemed to be. While the unit definitely appeared to me to be much more homey than what was portrayed in Imogen's mind, I do believe that those with memory loss can be subconsciously impacted by the places they inhabit. I do *not* think that they are in a state of indifference, especially in the beginning and middle stages of the disease. I have seen the visible difference that surroundings make on the mental health of a person living with memory impairment. I am a firm believer in colors lifting the spirits of those in a room. In fact, the mere act of posting coloring pages on the walls was noticed by Penelope. Bright hues are eye-catching, even for those whose brains are not operating to the extent that others' are. Imogen told me the story of her step-father who lived with the cruel disease. When he was in memory care, he happened to be completely *mesmerized* by a red clock that another resident had. He would always take it off of their wall and bring it to his own room. Because of this, Imogen eventually had to buy him his own clock and paint it red! My sweet resident, Elsy, would always point out how much she loved my bright pink and black shoes or golden hair. It didn't matter how tired she was or how often she had told me before.

I believe that the color of *personality* has just as much of an impact on the elderly. I believe that they *do* notice when one is happy to see them. I think that most people can agree that a merry, cheery heart has a profound effect on the quality of someone's day. This is the reason why it was so important to smile through the exhaustion just one more time. Smiling for *my residents*, the reason that I did what I did. As scripture says, "Heaviness in the heart of man maketh it stoop: but a good word maketh it glad" (Proverbs 12:25, KJV). One day, I came behind Grace's wheelchair making "vroom" sounds as I pushed her around real silly. Her response was, "Who is it? Somebody who cares about me." She knew that someone *that* dorky had to care about her joy. I had the choice to either go into work with dread or with a mission to make it a happy time for myself and those around me.

Each day, a new quote was posted on the residents' printed-out activity sheet. One day, an Irish Proverb caught my eye: "The light heart lives long." One of my residents once told me: "You are happy all the time. You have a great personality." I told her that I try to stay spunky. It's true; a light-hearted approach to life can turn many "offensive" situations into humorous ones. Taking my residents' actions and words with a grain of salt has done us all some good time and time again. I have found that this can apply to any relationship: "Good sense makes one slow to anger, and it is his glory to overlook an offense" (Proverbs 19:11, ESV). I believe that our culture has a habit of taking things too personally, too quickly. This can be exhausting. It has been so liberating to practice believing the best in others and finding compassion and humor amidst criticism and differentiating opinions. One day, I had a thought that I recorded in my journal: "Part of the human experience is understanding that all will fall short and mess up, and that it's not about getting offended, but rather saying, 'Ah, that's human.'"

In the memory care unit, it was oftentimes more of a challenge to get the residents to take a shower on their scheduled day than it was in the assisted living unit. Mrs. Leona was one of those residents who would normally refuse her cleanings. She would give a matter of fact statement of, "I don't think so," upon being asked if she'd like to shower. One day in particular, I approached her differently than I ever had before. After working at the facility for nearly two years, I had realized that my residents usually responded better to a fun, lighthearted, playful, and casual approach, rather than a commanding one. When caregivers begin to get argumentative, demanding, or to treat the residents as if they are children, the elderly pick up on it. In other words, I found that it is important to use the word "need to" very sparingly and infrequently when working in geriatrics. If I were to tell my elders that they *need* to do something, it would imply that I have a position of superiority over them. It would be like telling my parents or grandparents what to do. Those living with Alzheimer's and dementia are certainly not an exception. I observed the most cases of violence and opposition from our residents struggling with memory loss when they felt *further* stripped of their independence.

In Leona's case, because she had a good relationship with her daughter, I utilized her daughter's name as a familiar buzz word to encourage cooperation. "Lucy wants you to take a shower," I told her. When she would begin to say words that suggested hesitation, I would lightheartedly tell her that it was my job to give her a shower. I would keep the focus as matter of fact as possible, rather than making the task appear to be optional. The idea was to always keep working toward the goal of showering a resident as if it was *absolutely* going to happen. Sometimes, it was not achievable or even practical on that particular day, but I learned that it was something to go into with focused gentleness instead of timid hesitation. If I was not sure or presented myself as shy, the residents could tell and therefore would not trust my capability to help them. Additionally, it was important to make the harder tasks fun for the residents. The little ways that this could be done made *all* the difference in the world. When I successfully got my residents into the shower, I would quietly sing worship songs such as *Amazing Grace*. I would also ask them questions to distract them from the water, their complaints about how long it was taking, or how cold they were. Joking was another go-to for me that sometimes worked very well, especially with the more essential, mundane tasks. With Leona, when I told her to lift her arms up so I could scrub under them, I started singing the hokey-pokey. That got her laughing! In the same way, when I took Elsy to the restroom, I began to sing, "I'm a little teapot, short and stout," to which she continued singing the lyrics for me! On another occasion, when I couldn't find even one matching pair of socks in Elsy's drawer, I told her as I dressed her: "Maybe you've got a sock snatcher . . ." "That's not a very interesting thing to snatch." That got her chuckling! I adopted the philosophy that the best way to go about it was to make it fun; to make life fun! I loved to braid my residents' hair for the day, paint or trim their nails, massage their feet, do their makeup, talk about their marriages and pasts, sing while I made their beds, dance in front of them, or do projects with them. I believe that we often get out of life what we put *into* it. This applies to our jobs, passions, goals, and relationships!

In which you can ask yourself:

1. How can I have fun with my duty as a caregiver?

2. What is my word for the week (or month) that will define my demeanor toward those within my care? (Examples: soft, tender, kind, compassionate)

Chapter Twelve:

The Gift of Today

Dear Reader,

As a dear elderly friend of mine once wrote, may you remember that "God blinks, and one-hundred years flies by." May you remember that there is a gift to be found in every season of our lives. Allow the elderly to teach you at a younger age what they had to learn through years of experience: the simplicities of life are everything. As Ecclesiastes 3:1–2 says, "To every thing there is a season, and a time to every purpose under heaven: A time to be born, and a time to die; a time to plant, and a time to pluck up that which is planted" (KJV).

(Scribble 1) Aware of Lack of Awareness

"God blinks, and one-hundred years flies by"

The consternation that sometimes accompanies the last phases of life is a concept that I will not understand until I am there myself. I have witnessed moments of helplessness, where residents became aware of the fact that they could no longer remember things like they used to. They were losing a part of themselves, and neither they nor those watching could do anything about it.

One day, a resident named Nora approached the nurse's station with two pill bottles in her hand. She had found them in her apartment drawer and was frantically asking the caregivers and nurses at the desk if she was "supposed to be taking them all of this time." The nurse assured her that she did not need to be taking them and affirmed that everything was okay. Nora then had a break-down, crying and stating that she "could feel it," that she was "about to lose everything," and that her memory was going. One of our other sweet residents, Cicely, happened to be in the hall and approached the situation with a concerned look on her face. She leaned in real close to Nora to listen and comfort her with a hug. Cicely and I followed Nora to her room to make sure that she was okay and to console her the best way that we knew how to. Sometimes, an elder knows how to comfort their peers better than a younger caregiver can. They have been there; they are also riding along the ebbs and flows of aging. Cicely taught me a lesson that day: when there is nothing that I can actively do for a person, there is always a place for presence, empathy, comfort, and a listening ear.

There were moments in the Alzheimer's and dementia unit where a resident would make a comment that their memory was "getting so bad" or that they needed "a pill for their memory." These residents felt a change taking place within their body. However, over time, they transitioned into a stage where they could no longer distinguish between who they once were and who they had become.

Grace would sometimes sit in the community room and look up at the two-story staircase in wonder. She would be in awe of how I and others could run up the stairs with ease. As someone bound to a wheelchair, she understood how hard that would be for her.

Gregory was a young, wild soul within a body that struggled to catch its breath. He was a character, to say the least. One could find him flirting with the nurses, exercising on the facility's bicycle machine, or carrying a tune to a multitude of songs from his day. Oftentimes, the sound of a dog barking or a cat meowing could be heard echoing throughout the community room, and I would look up and find Gregory making the noises to stir up some commotion.

The other residents got a kick out of him and his unique energy. Yet, statements such as, "If only I were younger," were not uncommonly heard from Gregory. A young heart in an old body.

The elderly realize that, with age, they are losing things that they once had. That's hard. Any one of us that takes part in the human experience should be able to empathize with that. There was a man from another facility who would often call the front desk to talk specifically with our building's finance manager. I had the chance to talk to this lovely gentleman one day and ask him a little bit about his life experience. He told me something profound about his son: "One boy passed away, and *that's tough cause we're supposed to go before they do.*" You see, life doesn't wait for us to live it, and it doesn't always go the way we have planned.

I have learned that if I view each day as if it is my last, I can live in a commitment to my faith, my values, and not wait for tomorrow to find goodness. The verse in Philippians 1:21, "For to me to live *is* Christ, and to die *is* gain," has liberated me from the transitory worries of this life on multiple occasions (KJV). Every moment of each day is a calling to live in God and in worship to Him in *everything* that I do (no matter what it may be). As for my future, it is not in the control of my hands. I pursue holiness, and with it comes the liberty to not just survive but to truly live. As 2 Corinthians 4:16 states, "For which cause we faint not; but though our outward man perish, yet the inward *man* is renewed day by day" (KJV). If I truly have an eternal perspective, I can find eternity in every moment.

(Scribble 2) In Which Every Day is a Gift

One day, in a conversation with a peer, Charlotte said: "I've lived a good, long life. And I'm not worried about anything. And if I drop over tomorrow, that's fine. I've lived a good life. I'm enjoying every day, and if this is the last day, I'm pleased and thankful I've lived this long."

Similarly, Florida-Scott Maxwell wrote a book called *The Measure of My Days*, in which she records her experiences and reflections in her old age. She says, "Now each extra day is a gift. An extra day in which I may gain some new understanding, see beauty, feel love, or know the richness of watching my youngest grandson express his every like and dislike with force and sweetness. But this is the sentience by which I survive, and who knows, it may matter deeply how we end so mysterious a thing as living."[1]

Embracing the validity of this quote, it beckons me to ask the question of: "Why *now*?" Why does one tend to wait until old age to begin living life as a gift? I have come to the realization that humans spend so much of their youth *learning* that they forget to *exist* in the present. I learned that if I could grasp this concept at an earlier age, I would be better for it. I wouldn't always be looking for what's next but would approach the present moment with shock, awe, and appreciation that I'm even taking another breath. As someone who has spent most of my life struggling with anxiety, it is so important to remember that life is not at the mercy of my fingertips but is best left in God's hands and in His total control. I told a good friend of mine that the reason that I no longer fear death as much anymore is because I strive to live each day to the fullest. My goal is to fill each twenty-four hours with purpose in line with my creativity, with a servant's heart, and, most importantly, with obedience to God's Word as my foundation. The more I began to live this way, the more content and less anxious I became. I learned to surrender my moment to the Lord . . . and the moment after that to do the same. I will need a refresher on this for the rest of my life; my walk in faith is not linear but always leaves room for growth!

In which you can ask yourself:

1. What can the elderly teach you about the things that are truly important each day? Each moment? How can you live in response to that *now*?

1. Scott-Maxwell, *The Measure of My Days*, 90-91.

2. What would it be like to live each day in the light of your dying? Not for the sake of taking control into your own hands but in order to surrender, cling to His Word, and serve fervently?

Chapter Thirteen:

In This Body

Dear Reader,

I hope that this chapter reminds you of what a delicate task we are taking on when someone is entrusted into our care. May you see how caregiving comes around full-circle as a component of the human experience. The nakedness of vulnerability has been with human beings from the beginning of creation. Jesus is a prime example of how we can approach the weak of the world when their raw stories are cracked open and laid before our very eyes. I hope that these stories demonstrate what happens when we allow individuals the space to be who they are and behold their beauty as it unfolds. With the effects of aging, it is a gift to be able to give the elderly the token of caregiver reliability: someone they can depend on. That "someone" is you. May you know that love is a messy, unpredictable job, but it is a job that is always worth the risk.

(Scribble 1) To Babies We Return

It is ironic to me that humans begin this life in the innocence of infancy and after years of enduring the harsh realities of adulthood, return again to the likeness of a child. It reminds me of the scripture, "By the sweat of your brow you will eat your food until you return to the ground, since from it you were taken; for dust you are and to dust you will return" (Genesis 3:19, NIV). I have realized that humans are born with nothing and end with nothing but their soul. The body that worked so hard to grow deteriorates once again, folding in on itself; a box, opened for a moment only to be closed again and sealed.

I watched my resident, Maggie, endure the metamorphosis that life imposed on her. A human that grew to take care of her children once again became someone to take care of. Maggie was a woman that I knew to be full of spunk and sarcastic comedy. Even in her days living with the advanced stages of dementia, she loved to color, kiss her stuffed penguins (her "babies"), drink lots of coffee, sing along to oldies like "Purple Rain," and joke about the other residents. She would often reflect on her time as a hairdresser and all of the clients that she had in her earlier years. For nearly two years, I had the pleasure of knowing Maggie, laughing at her jokes, and hearing her refer to me as "little girl" or "little girl with the bow in her hair." Then, I observed her endure a drastic decline in health. Her consumption of food was at an all-time low, her words became incoherent (more so than they already had been), she grew terrified to stand up for fear of falling, and she went from using a walker to being confined to a wheelchair. It was difficult to see someone with so much character lose her bright personality. She was someone who brought liveliness to the community, and it was obvious that the residents and caregivers alike fed off of her energy. It wasn't long before Maggie became bed-bound a majority of the time, where she was changed, hand-fed, and would groan when re-positioned. She would bunch up her blanket within her hand and bite the buttons on her gown. She returned to a fetal position, her body curling in on itself, with her legs bent and held tightly together. Tender moments meant a lot to me, such as Maggie holding onto my hand as I fed her, singing a song as she looked at my fingers, or grabbing onto my lanyard to pull me closer and curiously inspect the keys hanging around my neck.

It was intriguing to discover that death often embraces the physicalities of those with memory loss in the same way that life embraces a baby in the womb of their mother. In a fetal position one is formed, and in a fetal position one may die. It was so essential for me to regard my elders as superior while also acknowledging the time-travel that they endured both in their body and mind. Walking into the locked memory care unit of my facility, the babies and bassinets within eyeshot forced me to understand that aging changes people. The toys that would normally accompany the desires of a child were not intended to infantilize the elderly. Instead, they were meant to accommodate them as they travelled back in time in their minds. Touching, admiring, and holding babies is a means of comfort for some individuals living with Alzheimer's and dementia. In fact, one of my residents by the name of Kinneth absolutely adored the little baby dolls that we gave him to hold. It was heartwarming to observe him as he would kiss on the babies, blow raspberries on their faces, and call them *sweetie*. One day, I decided to talk to Kinneth's wife in reference to this sweet adoration he had, and I was moved to hear that he had a multitude of grandchildren. Just by looking at him, I could tell that Kinneth was the most wonderful grandfather and that many children would benefit from his compassion in the world today. I understood *who* those baby dolls were to him. In his mind, they were tiny children in need of an abundance of love.

My residents that were living with memory loss would ask for their children in the earlier stages of the disease and would gradually begin to ask for their parents as the illness progressed. In their minds, they were mothers, then teenagers, then children, and eventually babies once again. Leona was a resident in the locked unit who would emerge from her apartment multiple times a day asking if her family had left yet, telling the workers that she was going home, and asking about her car. The only way that I could ease her mind was to say statements such as: "Your family knows you're here," "We're going to take care of you," and "We'll call your daughter tomorrow." Eventually, Leona began to ask for her *mother*.

Upon waking up one day, my ninety-four year-old resident, Elsy, asked me if her "parents knew she was here." In a similar scenario, while I was strolling Grace around the facility in her wheelchair, she mentioned that she looked like her mother and stated that her mom was "about eighty now."

Seeing my residents go through these transitions opened my eyes to the vulnerable child within us all – myself included. I had an epiphany one day as I observed the work that I had been doing for nearly two years. It led to a journal entry where I asked myself why I didn't see others with the same patience and respect in which I saw the elderly. This was during a particularly difficult time that entailed an abundance of changes taking place in multiple areas of my life. I have always been someone who feels the healthiest when there is consistency in my routine, and this particular season was anything but consistent. However, when my job as a caregiver collided with my struggles as a human being, I learned a very important lesson: if I could approach each relationship and season in my life with no expectations, as I did with the elderly, life would be a whole lot easier.

With my residents, I learned to not be offended when they said or did hurtful things. I understood that their actions were usually rooted in something other than a personal attack on my character. I discovered that life was so much more liberating when I approached each interaction with my Alzheimer's and dementia residents as if none of the previous conversations had taken place. This meant that each new greeting could be an opportunity for a fresh start, with endless possibilities for relationship. To apply this to my mindset has been a source of freedom in my life that allows for my friendships to blossom.

(Scribble 2) Aging Bodies

... *"so he got up from the meal, took off his outer cloth-ing, and wrapped a towel around his waist. After that, he poured water into a basin and began to wash his disciples' feet, drying them with the towel that was wrapped around him" (John 13:4–5, NIV)*

When I was first contemplating taking on my job at the assisted living center at nineteen years-old, those closest to me cautioned about the responsibilities of the position. I remember my family making statements such as, "You're not going to want to do that" and speaking on the tastelessness of the field of work. As someone that had been conditioning my heart to be in a posture of purity, I felt quite hesitant myself. Even the idea of seeing male bodies was a new and shy concept for me. The question circulated in my mind about whether or not I thought I could "handle" such tasks. Would it be awkward for me to bathe the opposite gender when I was not familiar with a body that looked different from my own? Would the older men make suggestive comments and put me in a position of humiliation? I was the girl who would turn my head during movies when one of the characters were unclothed. Yet, I knew that I wanted to help people, and I could not help others while simultaneously letting fear keep me from vulnerability.

Surprisingly, I came to realize that most of my residents were outwardly unashamed of their bodies. After getting comfortable with the newness of nakedness, I realized how natural the duty of showering someone and helping them get dressed had become. Body parts were just body parts to me, and we all have some. Showering became a normal task that needed to be done, and normal conversations could be carried out just as they would have if the residents were clothed. It reminded me of Adam and Eve before the fall: unaware of their nudeness and embracing the bare familiarity of being human.

However, in spite of this commonality between human beings, each individual's body is their own to possess. As a caregiver, I was given the responsibility to care for someone else's belongings. It was a tender subject that I was called to approach with gentleness. In *The Measure of My Days*, after Florida Scott-Maxwell has her gallbladder surgery, she states: "Finally the night began when my body belonged to brisk strangers. The ugliness of my age was exposed to trim, fresh women. I was at last sent to have a bath at five in the morning, and then more drugs, and the strangeness of knowing less and less until knowing ceased."[2] There is a kind of subjection to scrutiny that the elderly may feel as their bodies become foreign to their very eyes. Who they *are* morphs into a

2. Scott-Maxwell, *The Measure of My Days*, 92.

concept that they have to learn all over again. They have to detach from what they looked like before and embrace who they have become, in the beauty of life's transitions. I cannot tell how difficult that must be for them, and I will not be able to until I get there one day. I can only *try* to understand, as is the case with all efforts to sympathize.

One day in particular, one of my residents, Nora, had an accident on herself before she could make it to the toilet. I happened to walk into her apartment to take her vitals during that time and came upon the scene in the bathroom. It was evident that she was humiliated and didn't even know where to begin cleaning. I could have left and allowed her to use her physical abilities to clean herself, or I could come alongside her and alleviate the overwhelming burden, confusion, and shame that she was carrying in that moment. As I wiped her off, she said to me: "What a precious person you are." It was not about the kind of person I was as much as it was about being trusted with the tender moments of a person's transition into aging. I believe that glimpses of God's unconditional love are displayed when an individual allows it to flow through them in moments of vulnerability with another human being.

On another occasion, when I was giving one of my residents a shower, he told me to scrub his back really hard because he had warts that filled with dirt. Having suffered from a stroke, it left Leo with severe damage to his extremities as well as a limited ability to speak coherently and logically. While my first internal inclination at the mention of Leo's "warts" was a bit of a "TMI" thought, I reflected on this conversation later and was reminded of Jesus and the leper. Jesus did not shy away from the leper because he was "unclean," kicked out of the city, or spit on by others. He wasn't so prideful as to be afraid that someone would see Him interacting with the "least of these" and the mocked. Jesus got close to the man with leprosy in a movement of comfort, gentleness, and unconditional love. In the same way that the leper trusted Jesus with his shame, I have had the honor of being trusted with the vulnerabilities of the elderly. Human life is a delicate matter, but it is especially so when I can come alongside someone whose body is deteriorating in front of their very eyes. If the elderly can no longer trust their bodies, then I believe it to be essential for them to have someone that they can entrust their bodies *to*. One of my residents living with dementia represented this well. One day, he emerged from his room and told me with tears in his eyes: "I've lost my mind. *You can be my memory.*"

So many aspects of caregiving reminded me of Jesus washing feet. As scripture says, "He poured water into a basin and began to wash his disciples' feet, drying them with the towel that was wrapped around him" (John 13:4–5, NIV). The act of Jesus leaning down, the sacrifice of His time, His nearness to one of the most unclean parts of the human body, and the idea of drying feet with the very towel that was wrapped around His *own* waist. *Someone* had to be the one to wash feet, and it was the King of Kings that humbled Himself to the position of a servant. How could I ever be an exception to the calling toward such benevolence?

Indeed, I want to be the kind of person who meets someone and says, "Wow, someone just as imperfect as *me!*" We're all clay, constantly being molded by the Sculptor.

(Scribble 3) Daily Accidents

It didn't take long for me to learn that caregiving is a messy, unpredictable job – just as true love is messy and unpredictable. Choosing to have a servant's heart is choosing to get dirty physically, emotionally, and mentally and being okay with that. I learned that this choice is not one that should be made begrudgingly or coupled with constant complaint. It is to be approached with a back ready to carry the burdens of those around me. In Philippians 2:14–15, it is written: "Do all things without grumbling or disputing, that you may be blameless and innocent, children of God without blemish in the midst of a crooked and twisted generation, among whom you shine as lights in the world," (ESV).

In any relational commitment that I involve myself in, I realize that I have to be prepared for accidents in every sense of the word. Because of the fragility of being human, I have to expect things to go haywire every once in a while and not to get upset at the interruptions to my daily plans.

One day, a resident by the name of Tim informed me that he needed to use the restroom. Because he weighed over two-hundred pounds and had trouble standing due to a bad knee, I had to wait for my coworker, Liz, to help me. However, by the time I took off his brief and he went to sit on the toilet seat, black diarrhea exploded *everywhere*. My coworker and I looked at each other in absolute shock. The bathroom, my pants, and my work shoes were covered in fecal matter. The situation was so dramatic that I ended up calling one of my nurses to see if she could get a custodian in there for us. She informed me that it was *our* job to clean the area and that the custodian was only responsible for disinfecting. I called my college roommate to see if she could bring me a new pair of pants, but she was not home. You see, there is a time when you have to roll up your sleeves, put on a face mask, and get to work. There is no use in complaining when that same amount of time can be used accomplishing a task. Liz and I cleaned and laughed in both horror and amusement. We got the job done, because we looked at it as an obligation rather than a choice. We made the best of the experience and, weirdly enough, it was one that we bonded over for the sake of the absolute haphazardness we found ourselves involved in.

I have found a package of briefs in the freezer and a bed-pad in the fridge. I have found a bloody tissue with a signature on the bottom, as if it were a piece of artwork. I have seen a resident walking around with a shirt as bottoms, with arm sleeves hanging on either side of her after she "successfully" dressed herself. I have found a resident munching on a coworker's bag of pizza pockets and drinking out of another co-worker's drink. There are always surprises in servanthood.

In which you can ask yourself:

1. Can the person within your care entrust themselves to you? When they do, what will they be met with?

2. On the other side of vulnerability, we are often met with humanness. In what areas of your life are you hesitant to break through vulnerability in order to be more authentically *you*? How would your authentic self better serve those within your care?

Chapter Fourteen:

Outside of Caregiving

Dear Reader,

The goal of this chapter is to illustrate how an individual that is humbled to servitude can see beyond their own job responsibilities and into the equally-demanding responsibilities of those around them. They can understand that caregiving is not the only occupation in the world that requires much of its employees. This individual can see that their life extends far beyond those specifically entrusted to their care. Therefore, they will recognize that *every person they encounter* is someone to empathize with and love. A caregiver is not merely a job title; it is a way of life.

(Scribble 1) Do You See What I See?

There is more to an assisted living center than just the caregiving. It was good for me to get experience in multiple areas of my facility with job demands that differed from my own. In order to walk a mile in someone else's shoes, one of two things have to happen: you can either try *really hard* to intentionally understand or you can literally work alongside them and see what they see on a day-to-day basis. I was blessed to be given the liberty to do the latter. When I was first hired at my facility, I was trained to be both a waitress and a caregiver. Starting out in the kitchen, I could then look back as a caregiver and remember those disheartening beginnings that I had in the dining room: the nervous hands, feeling like I had to get every order perfect, being blamed when the food came out wrong, and being sent back to warm up someone's soup the second I delivered it.

Being a bingo caller on many weekends, I was able to see the competitive side of my residents. I learned which ones had an impatient demeanor and which ones had a laid-back personality. I saw the stress to get things "just right" for them and the kind of pressure this could cause. To call Bingo *just* loud enough, at *just* the right speed.

Working the front desk showed me a side of my individual residents that I didn't see when I was a caregiver to the masses. I saw which ones came up to the desk multiple times a day to ask the same questions. I saw the ones that got about twenty cups of coffee on a daily basis that I would pump for them. I saw the phones to be answered and the vitals to be checked every time a visitor arrived and left.

Getting a variety of experiences also taught me how job descriptions interlace. The impressions I had of the residents in the kitchen cultivated a shallow understanding of their character. I was inclined to only see Nora as someone who always complained about her cold soup, or Fay as someone whose food was never quite right. As a caregiver, however, the more personal, one-on-one care allowed for me to better understand *why* my residents were the way they were. It enabled me to understand that there were so many more wonderful aspects to their character. Looking back, this taught me that there is a whole world between brief interactions that can leave shallow impressions and the rest of an individual's life story. As my brother and sister's keeper, I am called to get to know someone's life and to not judge them based on what immediately meets the eye. As a caregiver, I have been able to practice the art of sacrificing my time in order to invest in what makes someone who they are. Come to find out, what makes someone who they are is an intricate web of life experiences, joys, and endurances. Because I obtained job experience in different areas, it made me a better caregiver. I was able to connect with those within my care on a deeper level, as I saw them in more than one light of life. May we always get to know individuals in the light of different hues; perhaps one color suits them better than another, and we will have the opportunity to see them *glow*.

Understanding that all areas of work intersect at one point or another also taught me how essential it is to move myself to empathize with other people's struggles. The importance of always being courteous to others cannot be overestimated; it will work in everyone's favor and create a better environment. It is so paramount to remember this in the midst of frustration and tension. I learned that *my* frustrations aren't the only ones that are valid. I could get into the mindset of always thinking that I had it the worst, when that was just not the case. When the facility chef was angry and conveyed that while making me a meal, I could understand that they probably had had many food complaints or special requests that night. My job was to be kind to them. It was also my job to remember that the same rule applied for my coworkers as it did for my residents: *there is a whole world between brief interactions that can leave shallow impressions and the rest of an individual's life story.*

In which you can ask yourself:

1. Who else is involved in your life and therefore impacted by your job as a caregiver? What is their story, and how you can empathize with their responsibilities?

2. When those around you are frustrated, can you pause and ask yourself why this might be the case? Can you take time before responding to think and pray? Can you remind yourself that your frustration is not the only frustration and that others can feel things, too?

3. What items are on the to-do lists of those you love? Maybe you can take time to ask them and enter into the head-space of what their tasks demand of them day-to-day.

(Revelations from Loss) Your Grief is Your Superpower

I was hit with the overwhelming plague of grief in October of 2020 as a result of losing my baby ferret, Panda. He was my little buddy; I called him my Stinky Slinky and Bug-Boy. As soon as I saw him at the pet store, I scooped him up and put him on hold. It wasn't until he passed away that I realized the impact he made on my day-to-day life. My schedule wrapped around his presence. When I first got him, I would often think to myself: *I just want him to be a happy boy.* I would wake up to him curled up in a ball on his bedding, let him run for a while before my college classes, feed him, clean his cage, and repeat the process about three times a day. The trauma of what Panda went through at the end of his life, however, made it hard for me to reconcile the good with the bad. Having gone through losses in my life but none that ever hit that hard, I finally saw how pain impacts the human spirit. When he died, I was wrecked to the core.

Trauma does that to you; it has a way of bringing to the surface everything you have repressed for so long. It unleashes the hurt so that you can heal. It was as if all of the struggles that I had gone through throughout the previous months of my life hit me like a ton of bricks. On top of an insurmountable amount of confusion related to how on earth I was going to process all of my mental health struggles simultaneously, everything was a reminder of Panda. I had flashbacks to the end of his life: a downward spiral of unanswered questions and hurt that I would never want a baby animal to endure. I struggled with the fact that I would never be able to cuddle him or kiss the little floof again. I would open my dresser drawer where he would normally be curled up in my clothes to sleep, and I knew that it would no longer be a reality. I couldn't put his cage away, the same way that a mother struggles to come home to an empty crib where a baby once lay. His cage and all of his toys remained in my room . . . and remained. I cried when I emptied his food and water bowl for the last time. I wrestled with the concept that humans are expected to move on with life when someone is no longer here. Why did that feel so much like betrayal? It seemed so unfair that life just doesn't stop for death; there was homework to be done, a job to go to, time passing by. Panda's toys still smelled like him; I would cuddle his favorite teddy bear and cry. I missed his little ears and knew in my heart that even if I had an animal again, they could never replace him.

I think that grief is such an uncomfortable feeling that we often fear it will overtake us completely if we do not push it away. I learned that it's important to *feel it*. In fact, sometimes the emotion is *so hard* to endure that we can't do anything *less* than feel it. One day near the end of Penelope's life, her son, Rick, called the memory care unit inquiring about his beloved mother. At this point, Penelope was no longer opening her eyes and was unable to engage in any kind of conversation. Still, her son longed to say goodbye – whether for his own soul or for the hope that she could still somehow understand his words. Positioning the Face-Time video so that Rick could see her laying in bed, I watched as he virtually had his final moments with the woman who raised him. "I love you, momma. I love you bunches," he said, sobbing. I couldn't help but wonder what Penelope was like in her younger years. Who was the mother that Rick knew her to be? Those final moments held a plethora of memories for her son. During that time, I was an outsider looking in. Surely, there was a depth behind that interaction that I will never understand.

Trying to push emotions away is not only unhealthy, but it's unrealistic. Loving deeply feels a lot like hurting deeply. Loving Panda left me feeling so broken that I wondered if it was worth it to ever get attached again. Yet, somehow, mourning made me empathize from a place that only the mourning can.

The day after Panda's death, I walked into work and heard one of my memory care residents crying from her room. I saw a couple of workers sitting on their phones in the community room and wondered why they weren't moved to compassion. I understood. It is scarily easy to become desensitized when one is performing the same job day-after-day. It is a never-ending cycle that can begin to feel hopeless and as if there is nothing more one can do for the residents' struggles. It becomes familiar, and the workers begin to feel numb. They are no longer shaken to the core with the newness of someone else's pain; the pain becomes ordinary and a way of life. I have been there, and that's the only way I can explain it the way that I am right now. I, too, am guilty. That day was different. The reality of suffering was reignited, and the rawness of being grounded once again *compelled* me to meet the crying resident where her needs were. I wanted to listen to her to see what she was trying to communicate to anyone who would listen. I wanted to stay with her until she was reassured that she wasn't left alone in a room by herself . . . that we were right outside the door. I engaged with her from a state of knowing that there are hidden hurts in the heart of every human. This very hiddenness can produce a type of loneliness that can only be eradicated with vulnerability between 1) God and person and 2) person and person. In order for that healing to occur between myself and another, I learned that I need to dig a little deeper, press in, and be attuned to the silent wants of those around me. Most individuals will experience the pain of losing their own Panda, and after what I have endured, it would be exceedingly insensitive of me to ignore or minimize others' suffering.

Through the loss of my little slinky, I also discovered why grief is known as a *process*. The guilt of what I could have done differently. The moments where I thought back to when I could have paid more attention to him. The anger at God; why did it feel as if I had concern for the preservation of Panda's life and the Lord didn't? Of course, I was reminded of God's great grace, and that suffering and death are a result of a fallen and broken world. Grief can be wrestling with God; crying out to Him. I believe that this, too, is okay. David cried out in the Psalms, Job cried out in his affliction, Jesus cried out before His crucifixion. May we cry out, my friends, but may it be to the Source of hope in the midst of despair.

The reason for writing this chapter was per the encouragement of a friend. In the midst of my passionate heartache during one car ride, I had some things to tell her about grief. She told me, "Have you written that in your book? You should." So . . . I do. The feelings that emerged from mourning made me realize something profound: do not wait until someone is gone to spend time with them, call them, or tie up loose ends. There is enough guilt that tries to creep its way into the grieving process. Therefore, it would do us all well not to heap up more reason for regret. It is easy to get desensitized in this world, to be self-serving, or to only cater to what is directly in front of us. Yet, when someone dies, we realize that it was only the little things that mattered all along. Like Panda sleeping in my dresser drawers or crawling up into my bed in the morning and playing with my feet under the covers. Embrace the little inconveniences, and *pursue* them if that means loving others better.

(Final Scribble) When We Kneel, We Learn: Remember Audra?

Remember Audra from the beginning of this book? Well, I believe that God allowed me to witness something beautiful when I saw her transformation over the course of one short summer. When I first arrived at the facility upon transferring to North Carolina for a season, I saw a woman who was exhausted, run-down, lugging around oxygen, and basically bound to a wheelchair. A woman with a strong sense of independence and courage that was begging to fully express itself yet struggling under the weight of discouragement. Just weeks before I returned to my home facility in Texas, I saw a woman who was no longer attached to an oxygen tank, was standing up straight, only using a walker, taking herself to and from the dining hall, and demonstrating a sense of self that was finally being retrieved. She was more positive than I had ever seen her, less aggravated, and kinder. Her sense of humor was no longer weighed down by negativity; it was as if the light that had always been there was finally allowed to show itself in more of its grandeur. When I looked at her, it made me happy and proud. Proud of her and proud of what the Lord had done. One day, she was sitting in her bathroom after I had given her a shower. "Sat up too fast," she told me, closing her eyes and taking deep breaths from the dizziness. I reassured her and said, "This too shall pass," to which she responded: "God can move mountains." That simple statement reminded me that no matter what we go through, how old we are, how young we are, or whatever circumstances we are facing, we must look at our God rather than our condition. About a week prior to me leaving the facility, I told Audra that she would be a beautiful poet. She had a way with words; a combination of both her intellect and her endurance through great struggle. I asked her what her favorite memory was, and she told me that it would take an eternity to think of just one. She said that she had many good memories, and for every bad memory and every time she cried, she had more good memories, still. That you can choose to remember the bad memories or to dwell on the good ones and truly live your life. She said you can remember the "sunrises" you've seen and "the times that daddy carried you home on his back." When she talked about her father, it was as if she was fondly remembering him, her mind temporarily transported to another time where his presence still graced the earth. A time when she could reach out and touch him, hug him, ask him for advice; a time when her laughs would echo from his jokes. Audra gave me great hope in the unlimited power of our God, as well as a new perspective on life.

(Dear Reader) A Conclusion

The beauty of this book is that it didn't feel like a burden to write. It didn't feel forced or inauthentic. It is a book that *wanted* to be written. My hope and belief is that a book that wants to be written will also reach who it wants to reach. Hopefully in that very reach will a spark of grace meet the hand, mind, or heart that grasps it. I am sure that there are flaws in this memoir as much as I am sure that I am flawed. I was not always the best caregiver nor are my tips fool-proof. The truth is, I will be learning all of my life; every dawn brings with it new discoveries.

Most of all, through this book, I hope that you see the heart of the elderly. I hope that you see their generosity. I hope that my words will be like looking into the eyes of a grandmother or grandfather as they tell you, "I care about you," while holding your hand in their own. I want you to know that *you* will not always be the best caregiver. There are times when you will fail. There are times when the day will feel big and the appreciation will feel small. Allow yourself to acknowledge those times as a part of the human experience, and keep leaning into *love*. I believe that we can feel hard things and still do the right thing. We can be burnt out but still strive towards excellence. We can yearn to know the souls of those within our care and meet their unique needs. All of this can only be done with the sacrifice of our time and the dying-to-self kind of love of Christ. I wanted to give caregivers the opportunity to see our elders in a different light. So often, it seems as if the aged are put into facilities and forgotten about. They are neglected, and their treasures are neglected along with them. My soul's hope is that this book has tugged on your heartstrings and given you a new perspective on the opportunity for a reciprocal caregiver and client relationship.

The job of a caregiver has the potential to be so abundantly more than just checking off a task-list. So much more than seeing residents as merely warm bodies. So much more than the hard times. It is about *leaning in*, looking beyond ourselves, and going the extra-mile in an effort to show the humans before us that they are valued and that their life-long efforts and contributions to the world have not been in vain. One can either be weighed down by the position or empowered and grown by the experience. The same residents that I showered were the ones that I shared laughs with. Because of that, I will always be able to cherish that time my resident Frank and I shared cookies in his apartment or when we held hands and prayed together in solitude. Isn't it amazing that a sanctuary of prayer can be anywhere? I will always remember him looking me straight in the face and saying, "I care about you, Kayla." I will always remember when he sprayed me with a shower hose multiple times while I was giving him a shower. He said, "Excuse me" after the first time . . . and then apologized profusely for all the times that followed. I will remember how I laughed about it that night, told him that it had happened before, and that it "cooled me off." I will forever treasure the last few times that I was able to hold his hand. I will remember the joy that it brought me to see those blue eyes flutter open on those final days. Every smile was a gift, then. Every squeeze of the hand, every touch. The precious moment when his daughter and I were on each side of his hospital bed, and Frank would look at me, reach up and rub my head, and then look at his daughter and reach up and rub hers. As hard as it was for him to speak, he still managed to get out an "I love you." It is memories like these that we can always cherish as a caregiver, as we see the profound blessing it is to share intimate moments and bonds with our fellow human beings.

The reason that the lessons in this book are presented in such a way as to hold geriatric caregivers to a higher standard is because it is necessary when considering what is at stake. We must understand that we are dealing with other *human beings* with life stories, feelings, personalities, perspectives, and souls. I believe that the more we are given in this life, the more that is expected of us. As scripture says, "From everyone who has been given much, much will be demanded; and from the one who has been entrusted with much, much more will be asked" (Luke 12:48, NIV). When it is someone's job to work one-on-one with others, there is a level of integrity that must be upheld, a mindset of respect, and a heart of compassion required. Yes, the job is *hard*, but that is why the expectations of oneself must be higher. I don't believe that it is ever okay to become lenient in the honor shown toward our elders.

Please remember, my Dear Reader, you can gain *so* much from working with the elderly if only you are *open* to it; if you are *willing* to learn in both the rich times and the strenuous. I believe that there is not one experience in this life that we cannot grow both from and through as individuals. I believe that life is not as much about how we feel as it is about how we *choose*. It is not as much about our circumstances as it is about how we respond to them. Perspective changes everything.

Sometimes we have to be comfortable with not seeing the direct effects of our labor. May we understand that our servitude is part of a mysterious eternal reality that is far beyond what we will ever fathom in this life. Sometimes, the very person that we have served will not remember that service a day later due to the effects of memory loss, but please don't ever think that means that the service is rendered void. In a mysterious way, it will forever be a kingdom reality. As one of my residents living with an advanced stage of dementia once said to me, "I have had so much fun with you. You made the people I wanted to hit, me not want to hit them anymore. I figured if you could be kind, I could do it too." *That* is what this job is about; making a difference in people's souls whether or not their minds will remember your actions. Trust the process and believe that the hiddenness of your good deeds will sow a beautiful fruit that you may reap in harvest time.

I have learned to kneel, because that's what Jesus would do. Jesus advocated for the least of these:

For the little children: "People were bringing little children to Jesus for him to place his hands on them, but the disciples rebuked them. When Jesus saw this, he was indignant. He said to them, "Let the little children come to me, and do not hinder them, for the kingdom of God belongs to such as these" (Mark 10:13–14 NIV).

For the prostitute: "All right, but let the one who has never sinned throw the first stone! Then he stooped down again and wrote in the dust . . . Then Jesus stood up again and said to the woman, 'Where are your accusers? Didn't even one of them condemn you?' 'No, Lord,' she said. And Jesus said, '*Neither do I*. Go and sin no more'" (John 8: 7–8, 10–11 NIV).

For the sick, when others passed them by: "'Who touched me?' Jesus asked. When they all denied it, Peter said, 'Master, the people are crowding and pressing against you.' But Jesus said, 'Someone touched me; I know that power has gone out from me.' Then the woman, seeing that she could not go unnoticed, came trembling and fell at his feet. In the presence of all the people, she told why she had touched him and how she had been instantly healed. Then he said to her, 'Daughter, your faith has healed you. Go in peace'" (Luke 8:45–48, NIV).

For the outcasts, who were thrown out of the city and deemed unclean: "A man with leprosy came and knelt before him and said, 'Lord, if you are willing, you can make me clean.' Jesus reached out his hand and touched the man. 'I am willing,' he said. 'Be clean!' Immediately he was cleansed of his leprosy." (Matthew 8:2–3 NIV).

I advocate *for the elderly*, because that's what Jesus would do.

I believe that when we kneel, we may learn something. And sometimes, that *something* is *profound*.

Quotes from my residents to brighten your life and open your mind:

(Memory Care)
Female Resident: "You stay out of trouble now, ya hear?"
Me: "I'll try to, it's hard."
Female Resident: "I know, but you gotta quit that. If you're gonna visit anyone at night, visit me."
–

(Memory Care)
Me: "Don't let the bed-bugs bite."
Female Resident: "I won't. I'll catch em' all and put em' in a bottle."
–

(Memory Care)
Female Resident: "I'm a little chilly around the edges."
–

(Memory Care)
Female Resident: "If I'd a known you were coming, I'd a baked a cake."
–

(Memory Care)
Female Resident: "I loved my grandma. When l started school, she made me five dresses so that I had a new one to wear every day."
–

(Memory Care)
Me: "I love you."
Female Resident: "I love you, too. Now why do I love you?"
Me: *laughs* "Cause we're sisters in Christ."
Female Resident: "Yeah, that's right."
we both laugh
–

(Memory Care)
Male Resident: "The military way. Hurry up and wait."
–

(Memory Care)

Me: "The people that are meant to be in your life will love you for you."

Female Resident: "I know that's right. My mother said that, and that was many years ago."

–

(Memory Care)

Female Resident: "Well, when we quit caring for people, that's when we're in trouble."

–

(Memory Care)

Me: "You seem happy."

Female Resident: "Well might as well be, because if you're sad you get nothin'."

–

Female Resident, with a grin on her face: "You know, they had to change me last night because I had an accident in bed."

Me: "Is that funny?" *I laugh* "Why are you laughing?"

Female Resident: "I'm laughing because I'm a ninety-eight year-old lady wetting the bed….oh lordy."

–

(Memory Care)

Me: "I'll be back."

Female Resident: "Where are you going?"

Me: "To the restroom."

Female Resident: *stares at me* "Well, that's one of the necessary evils that you have to do."

–

Me to Resident: "How old are you?"

Female Resident: "Depends on who you ask."

Me: "I'm asking you, missy."

Female Resident: "My daughter says I'm ninety-two but I don't believe it."

Me: "How old do you think you are?"

Female Resident: "Twenty-one."

Me: "Oh my gosh."

we both start laughing
Me: "I love my job."
Female Resident: "I love having you as a friend."
–

(Memory Care)
Female Resident: "I'm a daffodil, and that's important."
–

(Memory Care)
Female Resident 1 giving advice to Female Resident 2 when she
    was stressing out: "Why don't you just go on a walk and count
    your blessings? And maybe they're all squished up in a hole,
    but they're still your blessings."
–

(Memory Care)
Female Resident to Male Resident: "...Sit and hold each others'
    hand. That's what retired people do, isn't it?"
–

(Memory Care)
Female Resident: "When you get to be my age and things come
    along you say thank you, Lord, and if they don't you still say
    thank you, Lord."
–

(Memory Care)
Female Resident: "I think the more we give, the more we get."
–

(Memory Care)
Female Resident: "That's one thing you can do: take care of your-
    self. That's what mother used to say."
–

(Memory Care)
Female Resident: "I made it pretty good through school, not
    because I was intelligent; because I was friendly."
–

(Memory Care)
when I was doing her hair

Female Resident: "Just so it's out of my face, honey. I'm not looking for a husband, I'm just looking for friends." *laughs*

–

(Memory Care)
Female Resident: "Just check on me every once in a while. Stick
your head in and say, 'You okay?' And then you can go about
your business."

–

(Memory Care)
Female Resident: "I'm proud of you. You do a good job. And I
might just tell someone else."

–

(Memory Care)
Me: "Onward, said the fly."
Female Resident: "I don't think the fly said that."
we both laugh

–

(Memory Care)
Female Resident 1: "I'm going."
Female Resident 2: "Goodbye, I don't blame you." *laughs*

–

(Memory Care)
Female Resident: "Whatever you say."
Me: "Whatever I say. That's a lot of responsibility."
Female Resident: "Sure is, so you better say it right."
we both laugh

–

(Memory Care)
Male Resident, about his late wife: "When she died, I just gave up.
I tried dancing again, and it just wasn't the same."

–

Me: "How are you doing today?"
Female Resident: "I'm here."
Me: "That's a start."
Female Resident: "Is it? That's good to hear."

–

(Memory Care)
Female Resident: "I'm tired all the time."
Me: "You know, I've been the same way lately."
Female Resident: "Are you pregnant?"

–

(Memory Care)
Me: "Boys are tricky."
Female Resident: "Well, ya, but they're easy to fool."
Me: "They're easy to fool?"
Female Resident: "Sure."

–

(Memory Care)
Female Resident: "I hate to tell you this, but I'm leaving you. I'm
    going to bed."

–

(Memory Care)
Male Resident: "I just wanna go home. What's here is just patch-
    up, and I don't like patches."

–

(Memory Care)
while we were going on a walk together
Me: "What do you mean, jellybean?"
Female Resident: "They are not answering you?"
Me: "Who?"
Female Resident: "The jellybeans."
Me: "I was talking to you, silly."
Female Resident: "Oh, I thought you were hiding something."

–

(Memory Care)
Male Resident: "I'm just an old man, and I want to go home."

–

(Memory Care)
Female Resident: "I love when you come see me. Thank you."

–

(Memory Care)
Me: "How do you feel?"

Female Resident: "Oh, I feel like I'm too good for what I'm doing."

–

(Memory Care)
Female Resident: "This is my second job."
Me: "Yeah? What's your first?"
Female Resident: "Being a mother."
Me: "How old are your kids?"
Female Resident: "Uhh, the youngest is about twenty-one."
Me: "How does that work, since you're ninety?"
Female Resident: "I had them at a late age."
Me: "At seventy? I gotta write that down."
laughs
Female Resident: "It's unique."

–

(Memory Care)
Female Resident: "I like the young people because I can listen to
    them and kind of mother them a little bit."

–

(Memory Care)
Female Resident: "See, it's raining."
Me *laughs*: "It's not raining, it's the washing machine."
Female Resident: "It sounds like rain, does it not?"

–

(Memory Care)
Female Resident after I put her to bed: "If you want this house
    when I'm gone, I'll take you because I know you're a good
    girl."

–

(Memory Care)
Female Resident, rushing around the community room at eight
    o'clock at night: "Am I too late for breakfast?"
Me: "Oh *Resident's Name*, you're so cute. It's night time."

–

Male Resident to his wife that hadn't been getting around well:
    "Are you okay, baby girl?"

–

(Memory Care)
Me: "I'm writing a book."
Female Resident: "What's it about?"
Me: "Geriatric care."
Female Resident: "Wow, that's pretty deep."

–

(Memory Care)
Female Resident: "I was a hairdresser for four years, I could get anything out of anybody."

–

(Memory Care)
Female Resident offering for me to sit in a chair with her: "You can sit half if you want, because you probably don't even have half a butt, a whole butt, no butt."

–

(Memory Care)
Me, typing on the phone
Female Resident: "What are you writing, an epistle?"

–

(Memory Care)
Female Resident: "I've always been crazy, it's just working up to its full potassium."

–

Female Resident: "I was raised on plain food."
Me: "Potatoes?"
Female Resident: "Potatoes and . . . Yeah."
we both start laughing
Five minutes later, Female Resident: "Potatoes and beans."

–

Male Resident: "They say the most beautiful flower is the American red rose, and you're an American red rose."

–

Male Resident: "You're a honeybunch."

–

(Memory Care)
Me to Female Resident: "How old do you think I am?"

Female Resident: "About five."

–

(Memory Care)
Female Resident, about one of the other residents in the memory
    care unit: "How's grandma doing?"
Me: "That's your grandma?"
Female Resident: "No."
Me: "Whose grandma is it?"
Female Resident: "Heck if I know."

–

(Memory Care)
Female Resident trying to get her door open: "You have to be a
    contortionist to figure this out."

–

(Memory Care)
Me: "Okay, let me look her up (on the internet)."
Female Resident: "That's no fair, when I was your age we had to
    travel fifty miles."

–

(Memory Care)
Female Resident 1 asked herself out loud: "Am I crazy??!"
Female Resident 2 responded, nodding her head: "Yes?"

–

(Memory Care)
Female Resident when I laid on her bed and told her I was gonna
    go to sleep: "You deserve that. You gotta sleep every day, not
    just one time in every heck-of-a-day."

–

(Memory Care)
Female Resident: "And my legs are so fat, I used to have pretty
    legs. I don't know what happened to them."
Me: "Your legs aren't fat."
Female Resident: "They are, they're terribly fat."

–

(Memory Care)
Me: "What's the craziest thing you've ever seen?"

Female Resident: "It had to be something naked, I don't know."

–

(Memory Care)
Me: "When life gives you lemons, you make lemonade."
Female Resident: "That's right, honey."
Me: "What do you do when life gives you plums?"
Female Resident: "No I don't know, I don't eat plums."

–

(Memory Care)
Me: "She'll be coming around the mountain when she comes."
Female Resident: "Tell her to wipe the water off before she does .
     . . I like her."
Me: "Who?"
Female Resident: "Your friend."

–

(Memory Care)
Female Resident: "It looks like a Mexican car."
Me: "A Mexican car? What's a Mexican car?"
Female Resident: "Polished and shined to the nth degree."

–

(Memory Care)
Me: "This is a silly movie."
Female Resident: "It is a silly movie, that's why I like it."
Me: "You're a silly girl."
Female Resident: "I know it. That's why I enjoy living so much."
Me: "Aw."
Female Resident: "That's right."

–

(Memory Care)
Female Resident: "Oh me. I've laughed, my heart hurts."

–

(Memory Care)
Female Resident talking about her grand-daddy
Her: "He's just nice to be around. He treats you like a real person."

–

(Memory Care)

paraphrased, clipping Female Resident's fingernails
Me: "A fingernail just flew in my hair! You're gonna have to get the vacuum."
Female Resident: "Oh boy, I haven't used it in ages."

—

(Memory Care)
Me: "I think I've gained a few pounds since working here."
Female Resident: "Well, you look good. You look good for a few pounds."

—

(Memory Care)
Female Resident: "If I say I want to go home, I don't know what that means."

—

(Memory Care)
Me: "What are you thinking about?"
Male Resident: "You."
Me: "Why?"
Male Resident: "You're pretty."

—

Male Resident: "Excuse the silly comment, but if we were to get lost, you'd be a good person to get lost with."

—

Female Resident: "Please don't leave me."

—

(Memory Care)
Keys to marriage, according to one of my Female Residents: "You have to be flexible and remember it's two people from different backgrounds living together."

—

(Memory Care)
Male Resident: "Funny funny funny bunny."

—

(Memory Care)
Male Resident: "I wanted to see how fast you could run."
Me: "I can outrun you."

Male Resident: "I bet you couldn't."

—

(Memory Care)
Female Resident, referring to my pig-tail hair ties: "I thought
   they were ice cream."

—

Female Resident to me: "That's my girl."

—

Female Resident: "I love you Kay . . . so much. We're so happy
   that you're here."

—

Female Resident: "Rabbits are a symbol of Easter and they don't
   lay eggs. Now tell me how that came about."
Male Resident: "The rabbit I had laid eggs."
Female Resident: "You can go to hell for that, ya know."

—

Male Resident, making meowing and barking sounds
Female Resident: *cracking up* "Oh, you rascal."

—

Male Resident: "I'm always good. Look at the halo over my head."
Female Resident 1: "It's not showing."
Female Resident 2: "Did it fall off?"

—

(Memory Care)
*Female Resident, FaceTimes her son and sees his face on the
   large screen*: "Don't tell me that's me." *son cracks up*

—

(Memory Care)
Female Resident: "Life is just a bowl of cherries."

—

(Memory Care)
Me: "Do you want a cookie?"
Female Resident: "No, I want a hundred dollar bill." *laughs*

—

(Memory Care)

Female Resident: "Life is short. We have things that people has never said. You'd be surprised by how surprised you would be."

–

Male Resident: "Hey, sweetheart; you're great. I wish I were younger."

–

(Memory Care)
Female Resident: "I think we are past the point that a church is gonna help us."

–

(Memory Care)
Me: "We wanna know about you, *Resident's Name*."
Female Resident: "What do you want to know?"
Me: "Everything."
Female Resident: "I had crackers."

–

(Memory Care)
Female Resident: "That lady is so funny. She just came out of the refrigerator."

–

(Memory Care)
Me: "Do you want some ice cream?"
Female Resident: "No, I'm too fat anyhow."

–

(Memory Care)
Female Resident: "When there's work to be done, do it. And get a laugh in 'em. And they'll be back."

–

(Memory Care)
Me: "What do you think your talent is?"
Female Resident: "Well, I think loving people. I'm not an animal like that. But I look for people who need a little bit, 'You look nice today.'"

–

Female Resident: "We both have the same honeybug."

–

(Memory Care)
Female Resident experiencing memory loss, talking about her physical therapist: "I like him and he likes me, but sometimes I don't like him. It's nothing personal. I like to be friends before I like anything else. Maybe that's the old fashion in me."

–

(Memory Care)
Me, coming to get a Female Resident to take her to the potty
Female Resident: "There she is, that's my girlfriend anyway."

–

(Memory Care)
Female Resident: "I made it pretty good through school, not because I was intelligent, because I was friendly."

–

(Memory Care)
Female Resident: "No, I'm not gonna apologize for something that meant nothing."

–

(Memory Care)
Female Resident: "Well, that's enough of my preaching."

–

Male Resident: "Nobody's satisfied with anything anymore."

–

Female Resident to a coworker: "Thanks for spreading the sunshine."

–

Female Resident, with an open invitation to her apartment: "And anytime you get lonely, there's an open door for you to come on in."
"Honey, you are welcome to come into this room any time."

–

Male Resident, referring to the masks for COVID-19: "I hate these things; you can't tell if you're smiling or you're frowning."

–

(Memory Care)
Me: "How old do you think you are?"
Male Resident: "Well, I'm older than you, you can just put that on
    your engine. Last time I checked, I was about eighty-strings."

–

(Memory Care)
Me, holding Female Resident's hands to the restroom:
Her: "You have such little hands."

–

(Memory Care)
Female Resident looking at Male Resident: "Isn't he cute?"
Me: "Is that your boyfriend?"
Female Resident: "Yes."

–

(Memory Care)
Female Resident: *as she watched me break up her taco shell*
    "Your hands are so soft."

–

(Memory Care)
Me: "Do you like to look pretty when you go to bed?"
Female Resident: "Yes, you never know who you'll meet in your
    dreams."
both of us laugh
Me: "You made my day."
Female Resident: "Good, I'm glad I make someone's day."

–

(Memory Care)
*Female Resident opened up six packets of honey "just to look at
    them"*

–

Female Resident 1 about Female Resident 2: "She's very kind, very
    soft."
Female Resident 2 about Female Resident 1: "She's real slow but
    she's one-hundred percent."

–

Female Resident: "So many people here don't carry on a conversation and neither do I, so we have a strange time."

–

(Memory Care)
Me: "I'll be back tomorrow."
Female Resident: "We're gonna need it."

–

(Memory Care)
Female Resident: "What is this pill?" *Holding it*
Me: "Fish oil?"
Female Resident: "Fish oil?!" (After several attempts of not understanding me correctly)
... "Oh my."
Me: "It's for your hair."
Female Resident: "It's for my hair."
Me: "Yeah, it makes it golden!"
Female Resident: *to the other residents* "You take a pill this size every morning, for your hair."

–

(Memory Care)
Female Resident about Male Resident: "He's a sweet man. And I think it's natural. I don't think he's ..."
Me: "You don't think he's faking it."
Female Resident: "Nope. And if he is, I love it."

–

(Memory Care)
Me, closing the door: "Don't wanna give anyone a peep show."
Female Resident: "Let's do, it might be fun."

–

(Memory Care)
Female Resident to Male Resident: "I am getting worried about that tire around your stomach."
Male Resident: "It ain't bad."
Female Resident: "It ain't bad but it might be."
Male Resident: "I like it."
Female Resident: "If you like it, I like it."

Male Resident: "I'm not gonna do anything about it."
Female Resident: "And chances are you won't (do anything about it), but I don't care."

–

(Memory Care)
Me about Female Resident to Male Resident: "She thinks very highly of you."
Female Resident: "That's right, I do. His pretty blue eyes. And he can't help that."
Male Resident: "A guy's gotta shake it a little bit."
Female Resident: "That's right, you never know what's gonna fall out of the tree."

–

(Memory Care)
Male Resident: "I'm eighty-something. I don't know how far up. I'm gonna live until I die anyway. I'm gonna live until I die. Or until a jealous husband shoots me."

–

(Memory Care)
Male Resident: "Now I'm just an old man."
Female Resident: "What were you last week?"
Male Resident: "An old man. Just an old man getting older."

–

(Memory Care)
Female Resident: "I'm so full you could roll me."
Me, *laughs*: "You're so funny."
Female Resident: "Well, it's better to be funny than sour."

–

(Memory Care)
Me: "People don't look at you for your clothes, they look at you for your heart."
Female Resident: "Yeah, or your eyes."

–

(Memory Care)
Female Resident: "I'm happy as a bird in a tree."

–

(Memory Care)
Me: "What's wrong, *Resident's Name*?"
Female Resident: "I'm just sad?"
Me: "Why?"
Female Resident: "All of my little men are getting old."
Me: "Where are your little men?"
Female Resident: "Back there on the pot."

–

(Memory Care)
Me: "You are something else."
Female Resident: "Yes, I am. I'm a G-I-R-L, girl."

–

(Memory Care)
Female Resident: "I'm about to boil over."
Me: "That's supposed to happen, you're on the toilet."
Female Resident: "Well, we're right on schedule."
Me: "You're a mess.
Female Resident: "That's because I love my friends and
    neighbors."

–

(Memory Care)
I was praying before eating and a Female Resident mimicked me.
    When I opened my eyes, she had her hands crossed, her head
    bowed, and her eyes closed. When she opened them, she mat-
    ter of factly stated: "We have a lot to be thankful for."

–

(Memory Care)
We were carrying on a conversation and all of a sudden a Female
    Resident said: "Well, girls, y'all are gonna have to get me a
    bedpan."

–

(Memory Care)
taking Female Resident 1 to the bathroom
Female Resident 2: "I'm going too."
Female Resident 1: "This is a first for me."
Me: "This is a first for me too."

—

Female Resident, after I woke her from a nap: "I was in my dreams, sweeping a whole lot of leaves off of that big porch we used to have. I was working real hard."

—

Male Resident to Female Resident: "When you're growing up, you have no idea all that's going to take place."

—

Male Resident: "I wish you the best, Kayla."

—

Male Resident: "By gravy!"

—

Female Resident: "You are happy all the time."
Me: "I try to stay spunky."
Female Resident: "You have a great personality."

—

(Memory Care)
I held onto a Female Resident while she was sitting in the community room chair and she responded with:
"Where have you been? *I always need TLC.*"

—

(Memory Care)
Female Resident, talking about why she pushes her pager: "Every once in a while I get a little crying session."

—

(Memory Care)
Female Resident: "Now just give me time to think because I'm not trying to be tacky but let me tell ya, I'm popular."

—

(Memory Care)
Female Resident: "You see, the thing I get from you is enthusiasm . . . because you don't gripe."

—

(Memory Care)

Female Resident looking at a magazine: "People in the old days
are always just running around naked. They don't know what
clothes are for."

—

Female Resident: "I was tickled to death."

—

Female Resident as I was sitting by her bedside: "Most people
come in here and they just think about how they're going to
get out."

—

Female Resident: "I'm so glad to see you. You're one of my favorite people."

—

Female Resident: "If you were my daughter I would be blessed.
You're a honey, let me tell you."

—

(Memory Care)
Me: "How are you?"
Female Resident: "Terrible."
Me: "Terrible?! Why?"
Female Resident: "I feel so alone."
Me: "Come with me, no one should ever feel alone . . . how can I
be there for you?"
Female Resident: "Just be a companion, maybe that will help . . . I
feel so disassociated from everybody."

—

(Memory Care)
Female Resident: "I kinda got dropped out of a stream in the
middle of an ocean, and I'm sinking. Heeeelp."

—

Female Resident to me: "You're always in a hurry. Slow it down
girl, you'll get old soon enough."

—

(Memory Care)
Female Resident sleeping on the living room chair
Me: "I see one eye open."

Female Resident: "Uhuh."
Me: "Whatcha up to?"
Female Resident: "Checking you out."

—

(Memory Care)
Female Resident: "I think my hair looks pretty good today."
Me: "It does look good."
Female Resident: "Well, it does."

—

Me to one-hundred year-old, bed-bound Male Resident: "I see a
    handsome man."
Male Resident: "I see a beautiful girl."

—

Female Resident: "I'm so glad the holidays are over."
Me: "Why?"
Female Resident: "None of my family could come see me . . . it's
    just different. The only good thing about it was celebrating
    Jesus' birth."

—

(Memory Care)
Me to Female Resident: "You know it's New Years, right?"
Female Resident: "Yeah, I can't believe it."
Me: "Do you know what year it is?"
Female Resident: "Yeah, I think it's 03, isn't it?"
Me: "It's 2021!"
Female Resident: "2021?! Huh . . ."

—

(Memory Care)
Me to Female Resident: "What are you thinking about?"
Female Resident: "People that I don't like to."

—

(Memory Care)
Female Resident: "I don't want to go to bed. But I wanna sleep."

—

(Memory Care)

Female Resident: "You're as handy as a pocket on a shirt. That's what mother used to say."

–

(Memory Care)

"If I remember right, I spent three years, eleven months, and nineteen days in the Navy."

–

(Memory Care)

Female Resident toots: "You know what it says?"

Me: "What does it say?"

Female Resident: "Goodnight! Goodnight! Good gracious! Goodnight!"

–

(Memory Care)

Female Resident, matter of factly: "You're my best friend."

Me: "You're so cute! That made my day."

Female Resident: "Yep, me too."

–

(Memory Care)

Me: "We gotta fix that."

Female Resident: "You gotta six pack? That sounds like a winner; I'll come over and have one."

Me, *laughing*: "I said I gotta fix that."

–

(Memory Care)

when I was tending to her hair

Female Resident to me: "I don't know what you're doing, but I don't think I should go out in public with it."

–

(Memory Care)

Female Resident: "Who are you?"

Me: "Kayla."

Female Resident: "Kayla. Are you gonna be my guardian?"

Me: "Your guardian angel."

Female Resident: "Your guardian angel. Thank you."

–

(Memory Care)

In the famous words of Resident Grace, "If you like people, you work better for em.'"

Bibliography

Bible Hub: Search, Read, Study the Bible in Many Languages, biblehub.com/.
Scott-Maxwell, Florida Pier. *The Measure of My Days*. Penguin Books, 1987.

Made in the USA
Coppell, TX
09 September 2021

62113430R00085